The Green Unknown

Prepare Yourself for the Global Legalization of Marijuana by Learning the Basics

Wellington Z. Gupta

Disclaimer: The information contained in this book has been compiled from a number of sources with the aim of being as objective and accurate as possible at the time of its publication. It is meant to give the public an introduction to the topic of medicinal cannabis, and not to replace the expert advice of physicians or mental health professionals. Should you have any health issue or affective disorder that you think could be managed with cannabis, please consult an expert in those jurisdictions where marijuana is legal for medicinal use. The reader should have the habit of routinely let himself/herself be examined by a doctor, especially with regard to symptoms that may require diagnosing or medical attention.

The author or the publisher are not responsible or liable for any damage, loss, or disruption as a result of errors or omissions, whether those errors or omissions were accidental, the consequence of oversight, or any other cause. In like manner, they are not responsible or liable for misuse of the information contained in this book.

Dedication:

This book is dedicated to people who proactively seek to improve their physical or emotional health without giving up hope or feeling sorry for themselves. They somehow know that the answer is out there, and persist tenaciously in their quest to achieving their goal.

CONTENTS

5

Introduction

Thank you for purchasing our book. We believe that you will benefit by knowing and understanding the basic concepts surrounding marijuana as multipotential product of nature. The topics of cannabis, addiction, and the role that cannabis can play in addiction are so broad as to be overwhelming for those who are new to such subjects. This book offers a chance for anyone to become acquainted with these topics. The extensive contents of this book are the product of careful and deliberate research, which we feel has allowed us to put together a useful and quality source of information for the curious reader.

One of our main goals in creating this book was for readers to come away from it with a clear understanding of the role that cannabis has played in society throughout history. We take a look at how knowledge of this plant developed in different cultures, as well as what we know about it today.

This book presents an outline of the dramatic shift which has taken place over the last decade, and which is continuing at an ever-increasing pace, in regards to the acceptance and use of cannabis for medical purposes. We explore the popularity and effectiveness of using cannabis for a variety of physical and psychological ailments, with reference to the available medical research that has been carried out in these areas.

This book also offers the reader a solid introduction to the topic of addiction. In particular we take a look at hard drug addictions and at how cannabis may offer a potential avenue for their management and treatment. We present an honest look at what medical science currently knows about the efficacy of using cannabis to help those who are struggling with addictions to dangerous and potentially deadly substances.

The information presented in this book is intended to be expository rather than persuasive. We have not set out to champion any point of view, but rather to present research that may offer possible solutions for people who are facing certain health or addiction problems.

As you make your way through this book, it will be important to remember that health and addiction problems are rarely amenable to one-size-fits all solutions. This book should not be seen as a replacement for professional help, and any treatments you may become interested in should first be discussed with a physician who cares about your well-being.

If you or a loved one are struggling with addiction, then you should know that there are many resources available to you. Get in touch with a healthcare professional and stay open-minded about treatment options. Cannabis may be a good avenue to explore, as may more conventional treatments such as cognitive-behavioral therapy, which has delivered successful results for many people.

We've reached an incredible time in human history where we can find answers to virtually all of our problems if we are just willing to do our homework and research. Knowledge is available on a never-before-seen scale, and the search for truth can be a rewarding and life-changing experience. We hope that, through this work, we will be able to help as many people as possible find the answers they have been looking for and set off on their own journey of discovery.

Part 1: History of Cannabis Use

Cannabis During Antiquity

The developing social and legal acceptance of cannabis has been accompanied by a growing interest in how this plant was seen and used by ancient people. Researchers have now found that cannabis was used for a variety of purposes by the people of ancient India, China, Europe, Central Asia, and the Middle East. There has been disagreement among linguists as to the root of the word *cannabis*. Sula Benet, a Polish etymologist, postulated that its root is Semitic. She believed that the it evolved from the Hebrew word *k'neh bosem*, one of the ingredients of the anointing oil used by the ancient Israelites. In Hebrew, the word *kaneh* means "reed or stalk"; therefore, the translation of k'neh bosem would be "aromatic stalk." On the other hand, many scholars believe they are able to trace back the etymological source of the word cannabis to the Indo-European cognate *kannab*. Later on, it would have made its way into other ancient languages like Thracian, Scythian, Latin, Greek, and Sanskrit.

Thereafter, the word kannab would have become part of more modern languages like English and German. Kannab is associated with the cannabis plant used in the ancient world as a fiber and medicine.

India

The people of India have taken advantage of the medical uses of cannabis for thousands of years. Possibly the earliest reference to cannabis in the world comes from ancient Indian texts. Practitioners of *Indian Ayurvedic medicine* used cannabis as a kind of all-purpose tonic known as *bhang*. It was often prescribed to treat ailments such as headaches, upset stomach, insomnia, pain, low appetite, and sometimes even to lessen the pain of childbirth. Although it seems phonetically unrelated, the word bhang is thought to come from Sanskrit as well as the word *ganja*.

China

The ancient Chinese people were just as familiar with cannabis as their Indian neighbors. It was used as an anesthetic as far back as the 2nd century by a surgeon named Hua Tuo, who used to administer a mixture containing cannabis to patients before surgery.

The *Shennong Ben Cao Jing*, a 3rd or 4th century pharmacopeia, went into great detail about when cannabis was to be harvested, as well as which parts of the plant could be used.

Ancient Europe

In ancient Greece, cannabis leaves were used to stop nosebleeds, while an extract from cannabis seeds was prescribed as a remedy for ear inflammation. Meanwhile, the ancient Germanic tribes to the north consumed cannabis during festivals, possible to increase sociability within the group, which would have been important for ancient tribal societies. Traces of cannabis have also been found in Celtic tombs, but little is known about how the Celtic people may have used it.

Central Asia

In ancient Central Asia cannabis played a role in the society of the Scythians. The Greek historian Herodotus wrote that the Scythians took cannabis steam baths by tossing the flowers upon hot stones and "delighting" in the vapors. This shows us that, although they lived in widely different circumstances from those that most of us live in today, the Scythians likely used cannabis for many of the same reasons, such as to stimulate a sense of positivity and wellbeing.

Middle East

Several different papyri attest to the fact that cannabis was used over 3,000 years ago in ancient Egypt for medicinal purposes, particularly for treating sore eyes and lessening the pain of hemorrhoids. The nearby Assyrians began using cannabis around the 8th century BCE, and seem to have used it as a lotion. Cannabis was also used medicinally across wider Mesopotamia to ease swelling, stomach pain, skin problems, and many other conditions.

The roots of cannabis are irrevocably tied with humanity's medical and social history. Given these connections, it is no wonder that the laws which have attempted to rid society of this plant have largely failed. Much of what has been lost is today being rediscovered by researchers and ordinary people around the world.

Cannabis - The Medicine of the Middle Ages

It is interesting to see just how matter-of-factly cannabis was treated in the Middle Ages, when it was viewed as simply a plant to be studied just like any other plant. Physicians, caregivers, and regular people living from the 5th to the 15th century explored the potential uses of cannabis as a medicine, carrying on a tradition that had begun many centuries before.

Middle Ages in Europe

The prevalence of the use of cannabis during the Middle Ages in Europe is often attributed to the influence of the writings of Galen. The 2nd century Greek physician wrote that cannabis juice could be used to treat ear pain, and that eating hemp seeds could be used to promote a feeling of "warmth" and a sense of "well-being."

Galenic medicine was very popular during the Middle Ages, and may have prompted many herbalists to look into the various applications of the seeds, leaves, roots, and juices of the cannabis plant. An Italian herbalist named Dioscobas Tabernaemontanus, for example, wrote of a cannabis ointment that could be used to treat burns. Hildegard of Bingen, a German philosopher and writer, also wrote that a cloth with "cooked hemp" folded inside of it could be placed on the skin to treat a "cold stomach," and that open wounds and ulcers should be wrapped in cloth made of hemp.

Aside from the works of Galen, the widespread use of cannabis in folk medicine by the people of Eastern Europe likely grew out of ancient practices passed on to them by their ancestors. Cannabis was used in these areas to treat pain, inflammation, convulsions, jaundice, and even to ease childbirth. Furthermore, people living in Lithuania, Russia, and Poland would often inhale the vapor from cannabis seeds to lessen the pain of toothaches.

Middle Ages in Arabic Medicine

Arabic physicians and scientists during the Middle Ages also used Galen as their starting point for medical research into cannabis, and their invaluable contribution to the subject cannot be overstated.

Arabic medical writings from the 8th century onward delve into great detail about the various preparations and uses of almost every part of the cannabis plant. The first mention of cannabis in Medieval Arabic literature is as a treatment for ear diseases, likely because this was one of Galen's suggestions. Arabic physicians went even further, however, and wrote that cannabis could also be used to treat skin diseases, epilepsy, abscesses, inflammation, parasites, and even tumors.

Cannabis Use in Modern Europe

Europeans living in the Middle Ages were very familiar with the cannabis plant. Its seeds, leaves, and extracts were used in folk remedies across Europe, and a few of these remedies were even included in the pharmacopeias and medical texts of the time. Cannabis, however, was generally not given any more consideration than other plants which were also considered to have medicinal properties. This all changed as Europe moved into early modern times, when interest in cannabis, and especially in its psychoactive effects, took on an unprecedented intensity.

The Era of Exploration

Europeans sailed out of the Middle Ages by sailing off to explore distant lands. From the late 16th century on through the 18th century, Europeans explorers who visited places such as India, Persia, and the Middle East returned with fascinating tales of the ways in which these cultures used cannabis. The Danish explorer Carsten Neibuhr, for example, wrote in his book "Travels in Arabia," that the Sufi's of Yemen were fond of "raising their spirits" by smoking the "dried leaves of a sort of hemp."

Folk Medicine Revisited

Though Europeans living in the countryside had long employed the cannabis plant for its medicinal uses, stories of cannabis use in other lands sparked a renewed interest in cannabis among educated European society. Many texts, known as *dispensatories*, appeared during the 1700s, listing and legitimizing almost all of the old folk uses of cannabis as a remedy for ailments such as skin inflammation, burns, joint pain, dry cough, gout, incontinence, and low appetite. A dispensatory published in 1764 even recommended that cannabis be used to combat tumors.

The Era of Experimentation

When Napoleon's armies returned from Egypt at the end of the 18th century, many soldiers brought back with them a habit of using hashish. Stories of its psychoactive effects proliferated through French society, and writers such as Jacques-Joseph Moreau, Pierre Jules Theophile Gautier, and Charles Baudelaire extolled it as a substance that had the potential to expand the mind. Hashish shortly thereafter crossed the Channel and made its way into the hands of the literati of England, who likewise used it to enhance sensations and spur creativity.

Pioneering Work on Medicinal Cannabis

Burgeoning cannabis use among the thinkers of European society spurred a wave of interest into its medicinal properties among European physicians in the 19th century. One such doctor was William Brooke O'Shaughnessy. O'Shaughnessy noted that cannabis was safe to use, that it increased cheerfulness and appetite in his patients, and that it eased the symptoms of rheumatism, epilepsy, cholera, and tetanus. O'Shaughnessy's work was very much a precursor to the type or rigorous medical research that is being carried out on cannabis today.

The Interesting Interplay

An interesting pattern seems to have emerged in how Europeans viewed and used the cannabis plant into modern times. Historically, a curiosity about the psychoactive effects of cannabis led to an increased interest in its medicinal uses. It may be fair to say, then, that the psychoactive effects of cannabis have lead humanity to numerous other beneficial uses of the plant that could have otherwise gone unnoticed.

Introduction of Cannabis in North America

European society was acquainted with many different uses of cannabis by the end of the 1700s. Cannabis, however, did not grow naturally in North America, and the medicinal and psychoactive properties of the plant had to be rediscovered in Canada and the US many centuries later. Let's take a brief look at how cannabis was introduced into these two countries and how it eventually found itself on the wrong side of the law.

The Early Hemp Industry

Cannabis first arrived in the US in 1611. Various efforts were made throughout the following centuries to encourage farmers to grow the plant in order to provide England with hemp fiber to make fabric and rope. Farmers, however, generally preferred to grow more lucrative crops. Large scale hemp production came to an end during the American Civil War.

Canada was likewise tasked with growing cannabis in order to provide hemp fiber for France as early as 1606. England continued to push for hemp production once Canada fell under its domain in 1763, but, like in the US, was unable to garner much interest among farmers.

Growing Recreational and Medicinal Use

Cannabis largely disappeared from Canada once hemp production ceased, but it received a good deal of attention from American writers and physicians over the latter half of the 1800s. Various preparations of cannabis became widely available in American pharmacies over the course of the 1850s, and the effects of hashish were described around the same time by the well-known American author Bayard Taylor.

Interest in cannabis' medicinal properties grew in 1860, when they were cataloged in great detail by the Ohio Medical Society. By 1869, the periodical Scientific American had noted that "the Cannabis indica of the US Pharmacopoeia" was likely being used by some Americans for its intoxicating as well as its medicinal effects. Several poems, articles, and books describing the mind-altering effects of cannabis began appearing over the next few decades, such as an 1883 article in Harper's Monthly entitled "A Hashish House in New York."

The Road to Criminalization

Despite growing interest in the effects of cannabis among the American public, cannabis use was largely restricted to New York's Syrian community, San Francisco's Indian community, African American jazz musicians in New Orleans, and Mexican immigrants who fled to the United States following the 1910 Mexican Revolution.

Numerous racial tensions that existed in these areas at the time caused many Americans to come to view cannabis use as foreign and un-American. This led to a series of laws in the early 1900s which outlawed the plant state by state. Though cannabis use was virtually unknown in Canada at this time, Canadian lawmakers followed the international community and classed cannabis as a regulated substance in 1929.

The Swinging of the Pendulum
Today there is a heated debate going on in Canada and the US about the legal status of cannabis. Attempts at decriminalization began during the 1970s in the US and in the early 2000s in Canada. Though progress is slow, there does seem to be a steady reversal of the social and legal opinions that led to the criminalization of cannabis in the first place.

Notable Cannabis Researchers
Sir William O'Shaughnessy
History is full of mavericks and pioneers with the courage to challenge the limitations

of their times' mindset. Innovative people with the expectation of helping others surmount their frustrations and sufferings. The recorded history of medicinal marijuana has its own heroes. One of them, Sir William O'Shaughnessy, is credited with being the first to introduce the use of medicinal cannabis in modern civilization and even creating his own trademark protected tincture in England.

Born in the city of Limerick, Ireland in October 1809, Sir O'Shaughnessy joined the British East India Company (EIC) in 1833. The EIC was an English corporation that focused on developing trade with the Indian subcontinent and China. Sir O'Shaughnessy moved to Calcutta, India and lived there for about nine years. During his stay, he helped establish the Calcutta Medical College where he taught chemistry and medicine. Sir William treated patients suffering from various diseases and experimented with Cannabis indica. He found that this species of cannabis had the power to soothe and calm individuals with cholera, rheumatism, infant convulsions, and even rabies. It would ease their pain and, in the case of convulsive disorders, decrease the frequency of seizures. He prepared alcoholic tinctures of Cannabis indica based on native formulations. When he later returned to England, he marketed these tinctures under a trademark in partnership with Mr. Peter Squire, a pharmacist.

O'Shaughnessy writes that "in Hemp the [medical] profession has gained an anti-convulsive remedy of the greatest value" (O'Shaughnessy 1839). Nevertheless, he cautions that a rare form of delirium may be "occasioned by continual hemp inebriation," advising doctors to start with low doses. Indeed, high doses of THC have the potential to produce unpleasant side effects in people with low levels of tolerance to the substance.

Sir William was knighted by Queen Victoria in 1856, and some hold that she used Cannabis indica to ease her menstrual cramps.

O'Shaughnessy was a multifaceted individual. Besides writing a book on chemistry and being the first physician to use intravenous fluid replacement to treat dehydration caused by cholera, he developed and managed the telegraph service in India.

Unfortunately, there is not much recorded in regard to the last thirty years of Sir William's life. We only know that he passed away in Southsea, Hampshire, England in 1889.

Are there any modern, non-biased studies that show that the application of any active ingredients of cannabis have any positive benefit to the human body and mind? Is there any scientific basis that the ingredients of this plant can help the human condition? The short answer is that it is difficult to tease out the social, legal and medical issues from objective facts; there are so many studies with conflicting conclusions that no single "yes" or "no" answer can be presented. These questions have been considered, addressed and argued for more than five centuries. In fact, there have been a number of biologists, biochemists and physicians who have carefully studied the medical benefits of cannabinoids (the active ingredients of the plant). However, the fact that cannabis has been labeled as a "narcotic" in modern Western society has seriously hindered the progress of research into its medicinal uses. There were no such social or legal pressures in the past, and it allowed physicians to discover a variety of medicinal uses for cannabis that we are only just beginning to take a serious look at once again.

Although there have been observed benefits derived from the medical use of cannabis, modern researchers have attempted to apply rigorous studies to determine if, in fact, these medicinal properties are real from a scientific standpoint. These studies are based on observed, repeatable and peer-reviewed studies.

Despite the social and legal restrictions on the medical use of marijuana during the past 80 years, particularly in the United States, a number of scientists in the fields of biochemistry and applied medicine have made ground-breaking, objective studies of the effects of cannabinoids. Consider just these two "book-end" researchers, examples of the length and breadth of research into medical use of cannabinoids:

Raphael Mechoulam

Dr. Mechoulam is known for having done some of the first ground-breaking research on the biochemistry of the active compounds of cannabis, beginning more than half a century ago. A staff member of the Hebrew University Medical Campus in Jerusalem, Israel, he was the first scientist to have isolated delta-9-tetrahydocannobinol. He also identified the CB1 and CB2 receptors in the human brain, part of the endocannabinoid system. Over the decades, Dr. Mechoulam has also studied the biological reaction of human physiology to the various forms of THC and how they affect pain, appetite and inflammation.

Roger A. Nicoll

A professor of neuroscience, biology and pharmacology at the University of California, San Francisco, Dr. Nicoll researched the molecular receptors of the human brain and the reaction of the brain to the bioactive ingredients of marijuana, which he describes in his paper published (together with co-author Bradley E. Alger) by Scientific American. Far from being a "one-off" study, Dr. Nicoll's work has been carefully reviewed and studied by other biochemists and physicians.

In between these two researchers, there have been numerous scientists and students of biochemistry, human physiology and medicine who have investigated the effects of the various compounds present in cannabis. These include studies ranging from those described by the National Cancer Institute to such advocate groups as the Marijuana Policy Project.

Part 2: Legal Status of Cannabis

Should cannabis only be available to those who need it for medicinal purposes, or should it be available recreationally for all users? Should cannabis use be legalized, or should it be decriminalized? What's the difference between the two terms anyway?

The Debate: Four Perspectives

As we can see, there are more than just two sides to this debate. Let's take a look at the four main positions that are usually taken on the issue of what the legal status of cannabis should be:

1. **Cannabis should be illegal.** Those who believe that cannabis should be illegal often argue that cannabis causes addiction and harm to one's mental and physical health, or that we simply don't know enough about it to allow it freely into the hands of the public. They caution that legalization could result in more intoxicated drivers on the roads, or increase the chances of cannabis use by children. Perhaps the most common arguments for keeping cannabis illegal is that it may lead

one to try more dangerous and addictive drugs.

2. **Cannabis should only be available for medicinal purposes.** A slightly softer stance on cannabis is that it should remain illegal to the general public, but that its use should be allowed when prescribed for medical purposes. Proponents of medical cannabis point to studies which they argue have shown the efficacy of cannabis for treating pain, nausea, headaches, seizures, arthritis, skin problems, and many other conditions. They often contend that we still don't know enough to allow recreational use, but that cannabis use can be safe and effective when monitored by a physician.

3. **Cannabis should be decriminalized.** Many people who think that cannabis should be decriminalized argue that the war on drugs has failed and that people should not have to face criminal penalties for simple possession of cannabis. They view cannabis use as a personal choice that is no more harmful—or perhaps even less harmful—than alcohol or tobacco. Proponents of decriminalization also contend that persecuting the victimless crime

of cannabis use is a waste of both taxpayer dollars and the resources of the justice system.

4. **Cannabis should be legalized.** Those who support the full and complete legalization of cannabis often say that decriminalization doesn't go far enough. They argue that only legalization, taxation, and regulation of cannabis can take it out of the hands of the multibillion-dollar criminal drug industry, and that tax revenues from cannabis sales can be a substantial source of income for the government. They also assert that children are more likely to have access to cannabis if it is sold on the black market rather than if its production and sale is subject to government regulations.

The Debate Today

The overwhelming majority of North Americans believe that cannabis should at least be available for medical purposes to those who need it. Furthermore, the percentage of people in favor of either legalization or decriminalization has steadily grown over the past few decades, and today it is only a minority who believe that cannabis use should be completely illegal in all circumstances.

Current Legal Status of Cannabis

The legal status of cannabis is currently in flux all around the world. While it does remain illegal in the majority of countries, several jurisdictions have amended their laws regarding cannabis use and sale within the last several years. Let's take a look at the current legal status of cannabis in the United States, Canada, Mexico, Europe, and Uruguay. We can get an idea of the global trend in this matter by taking a look at the situation in these five parts of the world at the time of writing this chapter.

United States

The legality of cannabis in the United States varies from state to state. Cannabis remains illegal under federal law and in 23 states, but the federal government allows states to pass their own laws regarding cannabis use. Cannabis is legal in Alaska, Oregon, Colorado, and Washington, as well as in the cities of Portland and South Portland in Maine. The remaining states have adopted laws allowing medicinal cannabis use, decriminalizing personal use, or both.

Canada

Cannabis use for medicinal purposes has been legal in Canada since July of 2001. Though two-thirds of all Canadians also support the decriminalization or outright legalization of cannabis, the Conservative Party opposes any such measures. Nevertheless, several key court decisions have called Canada's cannabis laws into question. Laws against personal use often go unenforced, especially in the city of Vancouver. The Liberal Party has promised to legalize marijuana for recreational use by 2018.

Mexico

Personal use of cannabis and all other illegal drugs has been decriminalized in Mexico since 2009. Individuals are allowed to possess up to 5 grams of cannabis without risking criminal charges, the only stipulation being that they are at least 300 meters away from a school, a correctional facility, or a police station. However, individuals caught with more than the specified amount can still face criminal charges and steep prison sentences.

Europe

The European nation with the laxest cannabis laws is the Netherlands, though only in specific circumstances. The Dutch government takes a stance of non-enforcement for up to 5 grams of personal cannabis possession, and sale of up to 5 grams in "coffee shops." Cannabis use has been decriminalized to varying degrees in the countries of Belgium, Czech Republic, Denmark, Portugal, Spain, Russia, Italy, Austria, Croatia, and Moldova. It remains illegal and subject to criminal penalties in all other European countries.

Uruguay

Cannabis use has been completely legal in Uruguay since December 2013. The current law allows possession for personal use, home cultivation of up to six plants, and annual cultivation of up to 99 plants by registered growers clubs. Uruguay's newly elected president has stated that he plans to stand by the legalization of cannabis. However, he has also expressed "doubts" about the state-controlled sale of cannabis through pharmacies. So, while the people of Uruguay are currently free to use and grow cannabis, it is not yet available to the general public in the quantities initially proposed back in 2013.

Changing Tides

The past decade has been one of unprecedented increasing public support for the legalization of cannabis. Though in many instances, such as in Canada, the law does not seem to have kept up with popular opinion, there nevertheless appears to be a slow but steady worldwide trend towards the relaxation of anti-cannabis legislation.

Part 3: Biology of Cannabis

The Endocannabinoid System

The effects of the cannabis plant on the human body have been known, in general terms, for thousands of years. Whether the floral buds and leaves are ingested, distilled and applied topically or smoked, the results are remarkably similar. What has not been understood until recently, however, is the exact mechanism by which the bioactive ingredients, called cannabinoids, found in this genus of plants are able to achieve these changes in human physiology.

It was not until the early 1990s that researchers began to identify types of receptors in the human brain and, later, in other structures of the body, which were specifically triggered by cannabinoids derived from the cannabis plant. These receptors, part of what was later named the *endocannabinoid system*, continue to be carefully studied, and further research has revealed the complexity of this receptor system.

Receptors

In general terms, a receptor is a type of cell that reacts to external stimuli. The sensory organs, such as the eyes, include receptors that react to biochemical and bioelectric signals, transmit information, and cause physiological changes to other cells elsewhere in the body. In the case of the eyes, the cone and rod cells located on the inner wall react to wavelengths of light entering through the cornea. These receptors not only gauge the intensity of light, but also the wavelengths, patterns and changes in light. The signals the receptors send to the occipital lobe of the brain are interpreted as "sight," including brightness, color, and motion and pattern recognition. A far more decentralized sensor system is the skin, which reacts to pressure, temperature and pain; these signals are sent to the parietal lobe.

While these receptors provide the familiar signals humans recognize as the five senses, there are also other receptor systems at work in the body. These can "recognize" and react to other stimuli, such as *pheromones, hormones, peptides* and large *proteins*. When a specialized receptor is triggered by a *ligand* (a molecule that possesses an affinity for the receptor) and causes a response, that ligand is said to be an *agonist*. If the ligand blocks the function of the receptor, it is termed an *antagonist*. Either triggering a response or blocking a receptor's function can result in physiological changes. In some cases, these responses to a ligand may be immediate and profound, resulting in such gross reactions as nausea, rashes, altered perception, euphoria or other obvious symptoms. On the other hand, some physiological changes can be subtle, long-term and not immediately perceived by the person, including anti-inflammatory response or analgesic effects.

Endocannabinoid Receptors

The largest family of receptors is that of *G protein-coupled receptors (GPCRs)* of which more than 1,000 have been identified. These receptors are activated by molecules outside the cell and trigger biochemical responses.

In the late 1980s, research at the National Institute of Mental Health identified cannabinoid receptors in rat brains (Devane 1988). Human studies in subsequent years identified the cannabinoid receptor type 1 (CB1) as a type of G protein-coupled cannabinoid receptor, for which delta-9-tetrahydrocannabinol (THC) was a primary agonist. These CB1 receptors were found to be located on the surface of cells of the central and peripheral nervous systems and, to a lesser extent, the pituitary gland, thyroid gland and possibly the adrenal gland. When activated, the CB1 receptors modulated the release of *neurotransmitters.*

By the mid-1990s, it was determined that another cannabinoid receptor, named CB2 (cannabinoid receptor type 2), also existed. These receptors were subtly different, being chemically shorter in length and located in different parts of the body. Although the presence of CB2 receptors was also discovered in the brain, they were not as densely represented as CB1 receptors in that part of the body. Instead, they were much more common in the peripheral nervous system, immune system (spleen, tonsils, thymus gland, and white blood cells) and the gastrointestinal system. In his review of the endocannabinoid system, Parichehr

Hassanzadeh (2014) states that mapping of the CB2 response showed effects on neural plasticity and neuroprotection through the regulation of *neurogenesis* and *synaptogenesis*. In addition, proteins involved in immunity called *cytokines* (which also have a role in the inflammation process) are modulated when CB2 receptors are activated by their ligands. A surprising feature of CB2 function, however, is that THC is not its primary agonist. Instead, CB2 receptors are activated by *terpenes* contained in the cannabis plant.

Terpenes

In botany, a terpene is an organic *hydrocarbon* that makes up the majority of plant resins and saps. The term "terpene" is derived from the word turpentine, which is the distilled terpene from pine sap. Cannabis produces more than 120 different terpenes in the plant's *trichomes* (the same areas which produce THC). These terpenes make up 10% to 20% of the total oils produced by the trichomes.

These most common (and apparently the most bioactive) terpenes are borneal, caryophyllene, cineole/eucalyptol, delta-3-carene, limonene, linolool, myrcene, pinene, pulegone, sabinene and terpineol. The profile of terpenes (the percentage of each represented in a unit of resin) depends upon which cultivars (strains) of cannabis is studied; each has its own "fingerprint" of these compounds. To a lesser degree, other factors include the soil and water provided during cultivation and even the time of day when the plant is harvested (Terpenes tend to be volatile and can evaporate from the resin when exposed to higher temperatures.)

Cannabidiol

Apart from terpenes, there are at least 85 active cannabinoids present in the cannabis plant. One, in particular, has been the subject of a great deal of research recently: cannabidiol (CBD). As with other cannabinoids, it is produced in greater or lesser quantities in different cultivars of cannabis. It also apparently appears in direct and opposite proportion to THC: the more CBD present in a cannabis plant, the less THC, while high-THC cultivars have lower percentages of CBD. Unlike THC, the CBD compound is not psychoactive (i.e., it does not cause euphoria).

Oddly, CBD does not act as a ligand for either CB1 or CB2 receptors. It is, however, a very bioactive compound, particularly as it affects endogenous cannabinoids (those cannabinoids that occur naturally in the human body). CBD does this by directly stimulating the release of *2-AG*, an endocannabinoid that activates both the CB1 and CB2 receptors. It also suppresses *fatty acid amide hydroxylase (FAAH)*, which is an enzyme that breaks down *anandamide*, another endogenous cannabinoid; by suppressing FAAH, anandamide levels remain active to act upon CB1 receptors.

In addition, CBD is an agonist for the *vanilloid receptor* (since it also activated by the *eugenol* in vanilla and *capsaicin* in spicy peppers). These receptors are responsible for mediating pain perception, inflammation and body temperature. CBD is also an agonist for the *A2A receptor*, which has a significant role in regulating cardiovascular function, myocardial consumption and blood flow. It also acts, in high doses, as an agonist for *5-HT* receptors (5-HT are also serotonin receptors.), which confers an anti-depressant effect and has a role in regulating anxiety, appetite, sleep, pain perception and nausea.

Of great significance, it has been shown that CBD has a strong affinity for the *GPR55* receptor, upon which it acts as an antagonist (that is, suppresses its function). The GPR55 receptor is unusual in that it promotes bone reabsorption, which can cause osteoporosis. By suppressing this receptor, CBD can reduce and even reverse the loss of bone density.

Effects of Terpenes and CBD

Although research into cannabinoid receptors and their agonists is still in its early stages, it is already yielding promising progress. There is growing agreement that the GPR55 receptor acts as a cannabinoid receptor and may soon be considered to be the *CB3 receptor* (Battista 2012), which may further advance the understanding of the endocannabinoid system. As the functions of terpenes and CBD continue to be studied, their potential to modulate human pathophysiology may result in greater medical breakthroughs.

As stated above, terpenes act as agonists to CB2 receptors. Terpenoids (the chemical derivatives of terpenes) alter the permeability of both cell membranes and the blood/brain barrier, allowing cannabinoids to have faster and better absorption into tissues. The complicated role of CBD as a trigger in a series of signal cascades is only now beginning to be understood.

While it is still too early to predict specific therapies, some researchers are already compiling hopeful lists of possible areas where these studies can lead. Hassanzadeh (2014) writes that CB2 receptors, when activated, displayed the ability to affect mood disorders, movement disorders, multiple sclerosis, spinal cord injury, epilepsy, ischemic stroke, Alzheimer's disease, chronic pain and insomnia. Terpenes, according to Casano (2011), show the potential for treating immunosuppression, increasing cerebral blood flow, enhancing cortical activity, the ability to kill respiratory pathogens, provide cancer chemopreventative effects (that is, reduce the side effects of chemotherapy for cancer) and provide antimicrobial, antifungal, antiviral, anti-hypoglycemic, anti-inflammatory and anti-parasitic activities.

It should be understood that these are just potential uses of endocannabinoids in medical therapies. A great deal of research is still needed to provide any clinical uses. In the meantime, however, the humble cannabis plant has been recognized as a potential treasure-trove of beneficial applications.

Metabolism of Cannabinoids

In this section, we'll explain the most important issues related to the *pharmacokinetics* and *pharmacodynamics* of cannabinoids. These are two fascinating aspects of pharmacology, the science that deals with medications and drugs and the way they interact with our bodies. Pharmacokinetics studies how our body deals with the different substances. In other words, how it absorbs, distributes, metabolizes and eliminates them. Pharmacodynamics, on the other hand, seeks to understand the effects that those substances or drugs have in our bodily systems. There exist virtually infinite *metabolic pathways*. Each one of them is a set of biochemical reactions occurring in our tissues. A reaction creates products that, in turn, can become *reagents* and take part in the reactions that follow. The complexity of our body is unfathomable; no matter how much we try to make sense of it, it still remains one of the biggest mysteries in nature. The fact that everyone's metabolism differs due to individual variations in genetics and environment compounds its study even more and, consequently, makes it even more interesting. It is safe to say that no two people will be affected the same way when using cannabis. In addition, we need to take into account that the type and number of cannabinoids found in the different strains of marijuana available today varies, sometimes in a significant way. Their rates also change within a wide range. Some strains are richer in THC than in CBD and, therefore, have a stronger psychoactive effect. In contrast, others can have a much higher rate of CBD when compared to THC, so they can be used for their anti-epileptic effect sparing patients from the psychoactivity induced by THC.

THC is found in an acidic form in the plant, which is pretty much biochemically inactive. In order to become an active substance capable of producing its psychoactive effect, it needs to be neutralized. This process takes place by a biochemical reaction called *decarboxylation*. During decarboxylation, which is prompted by heat, the acidic THC loses a carbon dioxide molecule and, therefore, becomes neutralized and active. As it undergoes this transformation, the psychoactive substance's *bioavailability* (i.e., its capacity to be absorbed and become available where it is meant to cause its effect) increases. It is interesting to mention that, according to some studies, CBD exhibits the opposite behavior: As it becomes neutralized by heat, its bioavailability may tend to decrease. More research will be necessary to confirm this point, however.

Smoking has been the way that cannabinoids have been traditionally administered during the history of humanity. When smoked, cannabis is heated (and THC neutralized) and absorbed in a very efficient way through the large area where gas exchanges take place in the lungs. The effects of administering THC through smoking are felt almost immediately. After seven minutes of exposure to a source of heat that can raise the temperature of the plant material to 310 °F (154 °C), cannabinoids are neutralized. When cannabinoids are inhaled through smoking (or through vaporization), THC can be detected in the blood plasma almost instantaneously.

When cannabinoids are administered under the tongue or on the mucous membrane of the mouth (i.e., sublingually or orally), absorption tends to be less efficient. Cannabinoids effects will be felt within five to fifteen minutes. When ingested orally, the time required for cannabinoids to produce their effect can be roughly from forty-five minutes to one hour, and will vary according to the individuals metabolic characteristics. When ingested that way, although the effect takes longer to be felt, it can last longer as well. When cannabis is used as an edible product, cannabinoids have to be decarboxylated through the heat of a baking or cooking process. Otherwise, they will not be able to cause their expected effects.

After cannabinoids are absorbed reaching the *hepatic portal system* (a system of blood vessels that takes them to the liver from the digestive tract), cannabinoids are subject to a process called *presystemic metabolism*, whereby their concentration is reduced. After that, the blood distributes them to other parts of the body like the heart and fatty tissue. The brain gets a small percentage of the ingested THC (1%), but enough to cause its high. An interesting feature of the edible form of administering cannabis is the conversion of THC into a *metabolite* (a product of THC's metabolic pathway) called *11-hydroxy-THC* which displays a much intense psychoactive effect. This transformation takes place mostly in the liver, heart and lungs. Later, this metabolite is inactivated and excreted. On the other hand, CBD is metabolized by the liver and converted into *7-hydroxy-CBD*.

THC strongly binds to *plasmatic proteins*, one important one called *human serum albumin*. This fact makes THC's bioavailability (and, therefore, its effect) decrease as it becomes harder for the molecule to be distributed and metabolized. THC is not the only substance that binds to plasmatic proteins, and when it is administered together with them, they compete for plasmatic proteins and can displace THC releasing it to the bloodstream. Consequently, the effect of THC can become multiplied when other drugs are present in the system as it becomes free to diffuse into other tissues. After about 36 hours, THC is excreted through the kidneys and feces.

Now let's talk about what cannabinoids does to our bodies (their pharmacodynamics). The most noticeable phenomenon that takes place when the body is exposed to THC is what is called *post-synaptic receptors downregulation*. In simpler terms, this is a reduction in the number of receptors available on the cell membrane's surface. The density of these receptors is reduced and, therefore, the sensitivity to their ligands (the cannabinoids) is lessened. Consequently, individuals considered heavy users of cannabis may require progressively higher doses of THC to experience its expected high. *Tolerance* develops.

The development of tolerance is considered by physiologists a neuroadaptation as the body attempts to restore balance (*homeostasis*). This loss of cannabinoid power occurs for other biological reasons besides receptors downregulation. We believe that other mechanisms like *desensitization* (reduction of the capacity of the receptors to bind to the drug due to molecular changes in the receptor) and *depletion of neurotransmitters* are also responsible for tolerance development.

Part 4: Applications in Medicine

Does Cannabis Cure Cancer?

In spite of the fact that the federal government has considered cannabis a *Schedule I substance* for many years on par with heroin, state governments have been decriminalizing and legalizing marijuana, especially for medical use. The increasingly widespread acceptance of cannabis has been spearheaded by medical studies that have found it to be a tool in the treatment of pain and many chronic health issues. While many of these medical uses are backed by multiple peer-reviewed *placebo-controlled studies*, there are no conclusive studies that show that cannabis has any effect in fighting cancer.

Cannabis has been shown to be effective in treating certain symptoms of late-stage cancers (and side effects of chemotherapy) like nausea, pain and lack of appetite, and its value in these areas is inarguable. But many people are taking cannabis in the belief that it actually shrinks tumors, induces remission and even removes cancer cells from the body entirely.

If there's no solid evidence that cannabis kills cancer, how did this idea get started? Cannabis has been found to inhibit certain types of tumors in laboratory mice. However, the results of mouse research very frequently can't be replicated in humans. The gold standard of medical evidence is the *double-blind*, placebo-controlled, and peer-reviewed study. Unfortunately, there have not been such a level of research to study cannabis as a cure for cancer.

Countless scientific papers have been published addressing the connection between cannabis and cancer treatment, but to claim that this preclinical research is a proof that marijuana can be a cure for cancer can mislead people. Some of the studies have indeed found that cannabinoids can trigger *apoptosis* (cell death) and stop cells from dividing—cancer cells are characterized by accelerated division. Laboratory studies have also found that cannabinoids can prevent *angiogenesis* and *lymphangiogenesis*—the creation of new vessels and new lymphatic vessels in tumors, which helps the tumor grow and spread. However, human beings are much more complicated than mice. In some cases, studies have found that cannabinoids can actually prompt cancer cells to grow, depending on different factors like dosage. Therefore, mouse studies don't constitute solid proof, as THC actually accelerated the development of certain types of tumors under certain conditions.

Studies in laboratory mice are not the only factor that caused the belief that cannabis kills cancer, however. *Simpson oil* probably contributed just as much to this idea, if not more. Named after its creator, Rick Simpson, this oil is an extremely concentrated liquid made by processing pounds of plant material. It's very high in THC, the psychoactive component of cannabis that was also found to inhibit tumors in mouse studies. Simpson claims that the oil saved his father from death and even cured his own skin cancer. His claims were accepted because he didn't try to sell the oil. Being genuinely convinced that it was the cure for cancer, he began giving the oil away and releasing his recipe to the public.

The problem with Simpson's claims is that they are entirely anecdotal. It has to be mainly accepted on faith that, not only are these claims truthful, but that patients didn't actually undergo a coincidental remission that had nothing to do with the oil. It can also be assumed that more traditional forms of treatment that patients were simultaneously going through may have been more responsible for the remission than the oil was. It can be postulated as well that there were simply mistakes and patients never had cancer to begin with. Simpson himself never got a firm medical diagnosis on his skin cancer, by his own admission.

Simpson and his oil make for a great story, and also a beacon of hope for people struggling with a cancer diagnosis. Relatively uncritical feature stories in alternative weekly newspapers all over the United States added all the fuel the fire needed. People working at dispensaries across the nation have often blithely assured buyers that cannabis will cure their cancer when applied topically or ingested, even though this fact is something that hasn't been proved.

Since cannabis is a federally controlled substance, it is not so easy to get proof in the form of patient studies. The United States government keeps a cannabis farm at the Coy W. Waller Laboratory Complex on the campus of the University of Mississippi in Oxford for medical testing, but distribution of the product to laboratories across the country is limited and tightly restricted. Even in states where cannabis is legal, federal rules stymie research on cannabinoids. Universities that attempt to carry out cannabis experiments run into serious problems with legal sourcing; Buying illegally or growing their own could not only undermine their experiments but get them in severe trouble. Research laboratories can get their supply of marijuana only through federal approved channels and that can take a long time. Since cannabis is still widely in a state of illegality in most other countries, researchers outside the U.S. run into a similar logistical issue. Cannabis for scientific testing is therefore not forthcoming.

It is too early to claim that cannabis cures cancer. A lot more research is needed to clarify this assumption. Until these studies are conclusive, we need to remain cautious.

Cannabis and Immunity

The immune system is incredibly complex and protects us against diseases. It is composed of cells and elaborate biochemical processes that take place to guarantee the defense against pathogens and effectively eliminate anomalous cells that can develop into cancerous tumors. Scientists have discovered cannabinoid receptors not only in the central nervous system, but also in the spleen, lymph nodes, blood, and bone marrow of laboratory mice. All of these elements are involved in some way in the immune function. Consequently, the effects that the cannabis plant can have on immunity has been a topic of great interest to scientists around the world. They have been particularly concerned with discovering a way to understand whether cannabinoids suppress or enhance the immune response, and the mechanisms through which these processes take place.

Cannabinoids receptors are located in *B-lymphocytes*. These are cells produced in the bone marrow which then migrate to the spleen and other *lymphoid tissues*. There, they mature and become capable of carrying out their function. They are responsible for producing *antibodies* to specific *antigens*. There is some evidence that cannabinoid receptors are also found in *T-lymphocytes* and *macrophages*. T-lymphocytes are involved in virtually all aspects of the immune function and are the ones whose numbers sharply decrease in diseases like AIDS. There are two types of T-lymphocytes: *killer T-cells* and *helper T-cells*. Killer T-cells can scan what is inside the cells to determine whether they are infected or not. On the other hand, macrophages engulf apoptotic cells (cells that commit "programmed suicide") and pathogens like bacteria and viruses.

Scholars have been concerned about the potential of cannabinoids inhibiting the immune response and some studies have been carried out to study this issue. However, results have not been conclusive. The immune suppression elicited by cannabinoids has been detected in laboratories and not in human beings. Additionally, studies have been performed with very high doses of cannabinoids; something that is not consistent with practical settings. Therefore, immunosuppression is deemed by many experts to lack clinical importance.

Interestingly, some scientists hold that, if handled correctly, cannabinoids could eventually be used as immunomodulators and help treat immune diseases like *multiple sclerosis* and *systemic lupus erythematosus*. Nonetheless, to date, research regarding the use of cannabis as an immunomodulator does not have clear enough answers.

AIDS patients constitute one of the largest identifiable groups that use medicinal marijuana for various purposes like counteracting the side effects of HIV medications. Therefore, it is of the utmost importance to research the effects of cannabinoids on the immune system, as this group could be particularly vulnerable. Likewise, cancer patients often use the properties of the cannabis plant to ease the side effects of antitumor drugs like nausea and vomiting. Hence, it is of significant relevance to devote resources to research whether their immune systems could be compromised. As the legal environment grows favorable to the use of cannabis as a medicinal drug, such research should turn into a more concrete reality, and funds should become more forthcoming.

Cannabis and Inflammation

Inflammation is a natural response that takes place in our bodies when subject to a noxa (for example, trauma or injury, infection, poison, or an *autoimmune reaction*). It is the way that our systems defend themselves against those types of stimuli. Three very distinctive characteristics mark the presence of inflammation: swelling, heat and pain. When inflammation becomes chronic, as in diseases like lupus, multiple sclerosis (MS), *arthritis*, and *colitis*, then medicine needs to intervene in order to ease its ill effects. Inflammation becomes an issue per se.

As we know, CB1 receptors, when activated by cannabinoids, elicit a response which is mostly psychoactive. In contrast, activation of CB2 receptors has other predominant effects, one of them being the inhibition of the inflammatory reaction. This is a reason why cannabinoids that activate

CB2 receptors in the endocannabinoid system have aroused so much interest in the scientific community. As CB2 receptors don't exhibit a psychoactive effect, the aim of finding a use to cannabis plant independent of its psychoactivity has become a worthwhile target. CB2 receptors are found in the different body tissues and, when activated, causes cells to release less *inflammatory signaling substances*. These signaling molecules operate by establishing complex communication pathways between cells during the inflammatory process.

Studies carried out at the ETH Zurich/Swiss Federal Institute of Technology have confirmed that cannabinoids like THC, which stimulate CB1 receptors, are not the ones responsible for the cannabis plant's anti-inflammatory properties. On the other hand, they have been able to ascertain that it's the stimulation of CB2 receptors that eases the effects of inflammation through the terpene *beta-caryophyllene*, also present in marijuana. This substance is found not only in cannabis, but in plants like cinnamon, black pepper, and oregano, as well. And, by the way, recent studies have suggested that beta-caryophyllene could also be instrumental in the treatment of anxiety and depression.

In addition to these findings, studies performed at the University of South Carolina have found that marijuana has the potential to help patients suffering from autoimmune diseases, also the cause of sometimes significant inflammatory reactions. Autoimmune diseases can be very painful and sometimes fatal.

One known marker of inflammation in the body is the *C-reactive protein (CRP)*. It has been used in a study carried out in a sample of more than 9,000 people and published in the Journal of Drug and Alcohol Dependence. CRP blood levels increase when an inflammatory process is taking place in our systems. In addition, a high concentration of CRP in the blood has been correlated with an increased risk of cardiovascular disease. This study discovered that cannabis smokers may have a lower level of CRP than people who have never used marijuana.

As we are becoming increasingly aware, the environment where we live has the power to induce changes outside the DNA molecule and can also cause alterations in the DNA itself. Structurally altered DNA is known collectively as *epigenome*. This epigenome can be passed down to the individual's descendants. It seems that compounds in cannabis, through suppressing inflammation, can actually protect the cell from changes in the DNA molecule.

All these findings represent a ray of hope for patients suffering from diseases that are marked by strong inflammatory reactions. However, it is not clear yet whether—or how—cannabinoids could target other receptors as well and, therefore, activate metabolic pathways, which can be the cause of side effects. Future research will certainly help us answer all of these questions.

Cannabis and Analgesia

Analgesia is the relief of pain while someone is still conscious. There are pain killers for every medical condition, but sometimes a person's pain is so intense that conventional drugs do little or nothing to ease it. In a situation like this, a person might turn to medical marijuana to make good use of its analgesic properties. In fact, one of the most cited benefits of medical cannabis is pain relief. Scientists from all over the world have always been interested in researching its analgesic effects, and numerous studies have proven that cannabis can reduce chronic pains resulting from medical conditions such as cancer, arthritis, and multiple sclerosis.

Although scientific studies results have revealed moderate decrease in the intensity of different types of pains, there is no doubt that patients appreciate any reduction in their pain level. Several placebo-controlled studies have been performed to better understand the use of medical marijuana in the management of painful conditions like *chronic neuropathic pain* and pain from *rheumatoid arthritis* and related conditions.

It is known that THC can reduce pain, and some studies estimate that it has 20 times the anti-inflammatory effectiveness of aspirin. Cannabidiol is another significant pain relieving compound found in the cannabis plant. CBD can relieve anxiety, convulsions, inflammation, and nausea, and even inhibit cancer cells growth, according to studies carried out at the Department of Biochemistry and Molecular Biology at Complutense University in Madrid, Spain. CBD is believed to enhance the effect of THC on pain.

One of the most common uses for medical marijuana is to alleviate the suffering of cancer patients who are undergoing chemotherapy. There are various drugs that are prescribed to cancer patients, but many people feel no relief from nausea after taking them. Moreover, in cases of severe nausea, a patient can have difficulty swallowing a pill and keeping it down. Inhaling medical marijuana can be a solution to this problem. There have been many studies on the effects that cannabinoids have on chemotherapy-induced nausea and vomiting. In a 2003 study titled "Cannabinoids: Potential Anticancer Agents," Dr. Manual Guzman concludes that cannabinoids "exert palliative effects in cancer patients" by preventing pain, nausea, and vomiting, and also by arousing appetite. Many cancer patients swear by medical marijuana, saying it helps them with their pain where other medications have failed.

Another widespread use of medical marijuana is to ease the pain of arthritis. Millions of people are affected by it. It causes swelling, stiffness of joints, and pain. Arthritis makes difficult for people suffering from the disease to move their fingers or use their hands. Some patients are even unable to walk. The number one complaint of people who are suffering from arthritis is "pain," which can be never-ending. Medical marijuana is often used in these cases because cannabis can reduce inflammation and alleviate joint pain. Cannabinoids can treat *juvenile arthritis*, rheumatoid arthritis and *osteoarthritis*.

Multiple sclerosis is another common medical condition that can be treated with medical marijuana. Multiple sclerosis, or MS, is an inflammatory disease that gradually cripples the afflicted. In many cases, the disease ends with death. MS causes the victim to suffer uncontrollable spasms and neuropathic pain. Medical marijuana can alleviate these symptoms. A report from researchers at the University of San Diego in

California states that smoked marijuana is superior to placebo in "reducing spasticity and pain" in multiple sclerosis patients. It also says that marijuana offers some advantage over current MS treatments.

Cannabis has been used for medical purposes for many centuries, and though medical marijuana faces various levels of scrutiny and restriction across the globe, in-depth research proves that marijuana has analgesic properties. The excruciating pain that can be brought on by cancer or arthritis can dramatically lower a person's value of life and cannabis could be an answer to those patients.

Dr. Mark Ware, MD, professor of medicine at McGill University in Montreal, Canada, carried out a study with patients suffering from chronic neuropathic pain, which is characterized by burning or tingling, and is usually resistant to standard pain medication. Neuropathic pain still perturbs the medical community due to its obstination to respond to conventional treatments. It is thought to be linked to injury of the nerve fibers as a result of diabetes, amputation, alcoholism, back, leg, and hip problems, spine injury, shingles, chemotherapy, AIDS, and multiple sclerosis. The patients took three times a day for five days a single inhalation of 25 mg of 9.4%, 6%, and 2.5% THC herbal cannabis, reporting a decrease in their level of pain and an increase in their quality of sleep.

Along the lines of this study, Dr. Janet Pope, MD, professor of medicine at the University of Western Ontario in Canada, performed a meta-analysis that concluded that, although modest, there was a reduction in pain in individuals with musculoskeletal pain like the ones associated with rheumatoid arthritis, back pain, and *fibromyalgia*.

In 2011, the British Journal of Clinical Pharmacology analyzed 18 studies of smoked and orally ingested cannabis. Its conclusion was that cannabis was safe and modestly effective in the treatment of neuropathic pain, rheumatoid arthritis and fibromyalgia pains. Furthermore, the improvements in sleep quality brought about by cannabis helped with the treatment. It is a well-known fact that sleep disorders contribute to increasing the intensity of various types of pains.

Dr. Jason J. McDougall, Ph.D., associate professor in the departments of pharmacology and anesthesia at Dalhousie University in Halifax, Nova Scotia, carried out animal research to establish the effect of cannabis in the treatment of osteoarthritis. He found that sensitivity and pain were reduced by injecting THC into the joint.

Many medical doctors in the United States and Canada regularly prescribe marijuana for the treatment of different pains like the ones mentioned above, including pain in patients with cancer. They consider cannabis a safe medication compared to conventional painkillers like narcotics and other substances with also severe side effects, besides addiction and impairment.

For patients, the hardest aspect of pain management is the long-term treatment of chronic pain with opioids, substances like methadone and oxycodone. Medical marijuana can replace or, at least, reduce the use of these drugs in chronic pain management. Organizations like the American Academy of Family Physicians, the American Public Health Association, the American Nurses

Association, and (since 1997) the New England Journal of Medicine endorse the use of cannabis for the treatment of severe chronic pain.

Cannabis and the Treatment of Epilepsy

Epilepsy is a disease that can manifest in many ways. However, whatever shape it takes, it is a heartbreaking condition. It's a humbling experience not only for those who suffer from the disease, but for their relatives, and especially for those who witness the convulsive attacks experienced by the patient.

One of the most severe forms of epilepsy is the one known as the *grand mal*, marked by violent seizures and loss of consciousness. Grand mal involves the whole cortical area of the brain which becomes subject to abnormal electric activity; therefore, its name.

Other less serious forms of the disease exist, where epilepsy manifests itself in a more localized way. Abnormal electric activity is present only in certain sections of the cortex. For example, if the area that controls a certain limb, like the hand, is involved, only the hand will suffer from convulsions.

There is another related disease named the *Dravet Syndrome (DV)*. DV is an epileptic manifestation that affects mostly children. The onset of this disorder can take place when the baby is two or three months old. In general, the child starts suffering from Dravet Syndrome convulsions before his/her first birthday. Patients with Dravet Syndrome can experience 300 grand mal seizures a day, and it is linked to the mutation of a gene in 80% of the cases. As the child grows older, the disease worsens.

It seems that cannabidiol could be the answer to the ordeals these patients face. There is a famous anecdotal evidence in the state of Colorado where a strain of cannabis named "Charlotte's Web" (after the first known Dravet Syndrome patient to be successfully treated with cannabis) has been a huge help to treat people suffering from this condition. Charlotte's Web is very low in THC, the psychoactive substance in the cannabis plant, but has a high rate of CBD, which has proven to help preventing seizures. Patients with Dravet Syndrome have seen their epileptic attacks decrease from roughly 300 a week to two or three a month.

Dr. Edward Maa at the University of Colorado, Denver, has been carrying out research to determine which genetic characteristics make a patient responsive or non-responsive to the treatment of Dravet Syndrome through the use of Charlotte's Web.

In 2014, the Health Ministry of Israel approved a law that allowed the use of medicinal marijuana in children suffering from severe epilepsy. Children in Israel can be treated with cannabis in order to control epileptic attacks when they are severe and the patient is not responsive to other anti-epileptic treatments. It is a known fact that Israel is at the forefront of research linked to the medical use of cannabis. Although not legal for recreational purposes, dispensaries exist which are supervised by the government, where patients—with justifiable reasons—can acquire different strains of cannabis to help them ease their health conditions.

Professor Meir Bialer, a pioneer in epilepsy research and staff member at the

Hebrew University School of Pharmacy in Israel, holds that 30% of epileptic patients do not respond to existing anti-epileptic medications and continue suffering from seizures. According to him, cannabis might very well fill the gap.

AIDS Wasting Syndrome and Cannabis

As we mentioned before, one of the largest groups of people that use cannabis for different reasons are AIDS patients.

AIDS or acquired immune deficiency syndrome is a devastating disease caused by HIV (human immunodeficiency virus) that severely impairs the immune system of the infected individual. It mainly affects T-lymphocytes (or T-cells), which are specialized immune cells that are involved in almost every function of the immune system. Patients infected with HIV are vulnerable to various opportunistic infections and tumors due to their weakened immunity. AIDS patients experience severe weight loss and what is known as wasting syndrome or *cachexia* (pronounced ka-kek-sia). Wasting syndrome is not only marked by unintended weight loss, but also by muscle atrophy. In other words, individuals with AIDS progressively lose muscle mass. They experience fatigue and loss of appetite as well. Consequently, as their immune systems become extremely weakened and they continually lose physical strength, their risk of death and dementia also spikes. Thankfully, the development of antiretroviral medications has reduced the incidence of wasting syndrome in AIDS patients. Nevertheless, their side effects, which include nausea, are extremely undesirable. Depression and sleep disturbances are also commonplace in AIDS patients.

Cannabis can help this group of patients by decreasing nausea and increasing appetite. If the right strain is prescribed, it can lift their moods and alleviate sleep disorders. All this has been shown by anecdotal evidence, which has been widely documented around the world.

Despite these benefits, there are still some concerns in regard to the effect of cannabis on the immunity of patients with AIDS. More research is needed to be able to guarantee that cannabis does not suppress immunity and, therefore, does not make these patients more vulnerable to opportunistic infections and tumors. Consequently, it is of utmost importance that patients who wish to explore the option of using cannabis as a way to ease the ailments tied to the disease work side-by-side with a physician knowledgeable and experienced in treating AIDS-related issues with cannabis medication so as to prevent long-term harm.

Cannabis in the Management, Treatment, and Prevention of Diabetes

Diabetes mellitus a group of metabolic diseases characterized by the body's inability to absorb glucose from the blood. Over time, elevated blood sugar levels can lead to other health complications, such as chronic kidney failure, stroke, and cardiovascular disease. Since the early 2000s researchers have begun looking at the possible use of cannabis for the management, treatment, and prevention of diabetes. The results to date seem to suggest that it can have benefits in all three areas.

One of the first studies to be done on cannabis and diabetes found that cannabinoids were very effective in lessening the pain of diabetic neuropathy, a nerve disorder caused by diabetes (Dogrul et al. 2004). Another paper, published in 2006, concluded that cannabinoids were also useful in the treatment of an ocular disease known as diabetic retinopathy because they decreased inflammation and neurotoxicity (El-Remessy et al.). The anti-oxidative and anti-inflammatory effects of cannabinoids have furthermore been found to attenuate the cardiac dysfunction which occurs in a disorder known as diabetic cardiomyopathy (Rajesh et al. 2010).

An early study to look at if cannabinoid could help prevent diabetes, which was carried out on mice, found that the cannabinoid cannabidiol not only delayed the onset of diabetes, but in many cases prevented it altogether (Weiss et al. 2006). A cross-sectional, 2012 study with a sample size of 10,896 adults showed that cannabis use was associated with a lower rate of diabetes in humans as well (Rajavashisth et al. 2012). These results were reinforced in a 2013 paper which found that cannabis users showed lower fasting insulin levels and tended to have a smaller waist circumference (Penner, Buettner, and Mittleman).

Perhaps the strongest evidence to be published so far for the argument that cannabis can help prevent the onset of diabetes was a 2015 meta-analysis in which the authors gathered together data on cannabis and diabetes from eight different national surveys (Alshaarawy and Anthony). They concluded that "cannabis smoking and diabetes mellitus are inversely associated" and suggested that there was now a stable evidence base for clinical research on the subject.

So it seems that cannabis use is associated with a decreased chance of developing diabetes, but can it be used to treat diabetes in individuals who already have it? While there hasn't been much research in this area, one interesting 2013 study did take a look at using the cannabinoid known as tetrahydrocannabivarin (THCV) to treat type 2 diabetes in mice (Wargent et al.), with very promising results. Because THCV increased insulin sensitivity, the researchers concluded that "THCV is a new potential treatment against   obesity-associated   glucose intolerance."

Given the infancy of cannabis research as a whole, it is encouraging to see how much is already known about cannabis and diabetes. The medical community can hopefully build on this pioneering work in order to come up with effective models of diabetes treatment and symptom management using cannabis.

Short- and Long-Term Side Effects

Receptors, when activated, elicit physiological responses. However, those same receptors (which have molecular specificity to the drugs they bind to) are not only present on the membranes of the cells in the tissues we need to target; they can also be found in other tissues we would rather leave unaffected. And that is one of the reasons that substances like THC can produce different side effects.

In the specific case of cannabinoids, it is thought that side effects are mostly linked to THC and not to CBD. As a matter of fact, CBD would help counteract the adverse effects of THC, which usually appear when high doses of this cannabinoid are consumed.

We will describe two categories of undesirable effects: short- and long-term.

Short-Term Side Effects

A common adverse reaction to THC is postural orthostatic hypotension, which is characterized by giddiness experienced when the individual rises after being in a reclined position. Therefore, it is important to consider this when under the effects of THC in order to prevent falls, especially in older people. In addition, blood pressure tends to rise, which is also a risk factor that can lead to stroke or *ministrokes* (also known as *transient ischemic attacks)* in susceptible individuals. *Tachycardia* (a heartbeat in excess of 100 beats per minute) is an adverse reaction of THC consumption that also needs to be taken into consideration. People with cardiovascular conditions may be more vulnerable to heart attacks.

A new issue that physicians are becoming aware of is *cannabinoid hyperemesis syndrome*, which is mostly characterized by nausea and vomiting.

In addition to these negative physiological reactions to the use of THC, high doses of the drug can have very unpleasant psychiatric effects marked by *paranoia* and *hallucination*, which, in general, subside after a few hours.

The good news is that there are very few cannabis receptors in the respiratory center of the brain stem, which is where movements of the diaphragm and other respiratory muscles are regulated. Consequently, there's no risk of *respiratory arrest* as in the case of opioids overdose. Some experts estimate that an individual would need to smoke roughly 1,500 pounds of marijuana during fifteen minutes for the drug to have a lethal effect.

Long-Term Side Effects

As far as long-term side effects are concerned, the product of the combustion process that takes place when the cannabis plant is smoked can be the cause of irritation of the *mucous membrane* that lines the lungs. This can eventually lead to *chronic bronchitis*, which can be prevented by using other delivery methods as will be explained further on in the book.

In terms of cognition, medical literature describes problems tied to impairment of intellectual executive functions like planning, reasoning, and the use of working memory. It is generally accepted that these effects are reversible after discontinuing the use of marijuana.

Moreover, some experts suggest that cannabis can trigger the onset of *schizophrenia* and *psychosis* in individuals genetically predisposed to this disorder. Nonetheless, this risk decreases as the person ages and his/her nervous system matures.

Finally, it is important to stress that marijuana consumption can increase the risk of heart attack and stroke in especially susceptible individuals. The use of strains with higher concentrations of CBD and lower rates of THC could help prevent these issues. However, we need to keep in mind that the use of any cannabis strain needs to be supervised by an expert physician.

Part 5: Species of Marijuana

Marijuana is a plant that is little understood outside of the industry, and many of the terms that are used to describe it can seem cryptic to those unfamiliar with it. The plant is actually comprised of three distinct species with different observable physical characteristics and chemical features. The most known species of cannabis are *indica* and *sativa*, but there is, in addition, a third type known as *ruderalis*. Each of these three species has their own specific uses, which are different from their kin.

Cannabis Indica

Folk history and the distribution patterns of the cannabis species indicate that all of it descends from Cannabis indica. This type developed, first naturally then agriculturally, in South Central Asia in places like modern-day India, Pakistan, and Afghanistan. It is known for its unique growth pattern, which is straight up like a pine. Its leaves are broad and have a dark-green color. It produces massive cola buds and is known for being extremely potent. Its effects are strong and body-centric, resulting in a high that can leave those unfamiliar with the strains stuck to their couch. It is useful for people suffering from chronic pain. Common strains include Afghani, Hindu Kush, Medicine Man, Warlock, and Grand Daddy Purple.

Cannabis Sativa

Cannabis sativa is a strain that was developed from indica strains hundreds of years ago. When Cannabis indica was carried from the old world to the new after Columbus, it set the stage for the creation of this new species in what it is today Mexico and Colombia. It is also originary from Thailand and South East Asia. Since the environmental and cultural factors surrounding the plant were different, it eventually became easy to discern differences from its parent. Sativas, rather than growing straight like a tree, grow more like bushes. There is a central trunk, but it has many branches that are long and full of leaves, which are narrow and have a light-green color. Chemically speaking, it brings about a more cerebral high, which means it produces all the positive medicinal effects without the sluggishness that comes with using indicas. The strains in this category tend to be used by people that need to be active and not have secondary psychoactive effects get in the way of a daily routine. Some of the more popular or well-known strains are Sour Diesel, Haze, and Maui Waui.

Cannabis Ruderalis

Cannabis ruderalis was developed in Northern Asia, and it is far more similar to industrial hemp than the other two. THC content is generally very low, often not having enough even to impart a psychoactive effect. The most useful aspects of this unusual species are just how fast it is ready to be harvested and how hardy it is. Since it developed in harsh climates with limited growing seasons, it finishes much faster than any other species of cannabis and makes much better use of soil nutrients. It produces far more woody stems and fewer flowers than other plants, making it ideal for industrial use. Given the longstanding prohibition on industrial hemp in the United States, ruderalis is often unknown even to enthusiasts. It has, however, been crossbred with indicas and sativas to create fast, auto-flowering plants that can be cropped in a month and a half or less. Ruderalis was used to create the flowering properties of the strain known as B.C. Big Bud, or colloquially Beasters. Other strains of the species are Automatic AK-47, Mighty Mite, and Ruderalis Skunk.

Times are changing, and sentiment regarding cannabis is becoming increasingly positive. States are pushing for hemp farming again, and the medical marijuana industry is showing no signs of slowing its growth anytime soon. Understanding the different strains and their places within the greater market can help get the most of the changing litigation and culture. It can also be useful to deal with a medical issue that requires marijuana as a remedy, since the ideal uses are so different.

When we combine strains, we obtain hybrids, whose effect is linked to the proportion of cannabinoids that each strain contains. Combining sativa and indica will result in strains characterized by having properties belonging to both species. The famous Charlotte's Web is a hybrid strain created as a result of the combination of a strain of Cannabis indica with another of Cannabis ruderalis, this latter having a very low concentration of psychoactive cannabinoids. The resulting strain has a large percentage of CNB (Cannabidiol), cannabinoid known to have anti-epileptic effects.

Part 6: Delivery Methods

Medical cannabis works differently in each individual, and this is also true when considering the delivery method chosen by the person. Intensity and duration are two variables that depend on everyone's metabolism and particular circumstances.

Smoking and Vaporization

Smoked cannabis has always been the most traditional way marijuana has been consumed in the history of humanity. Hemp leaves or flowers are dried and then smoked with a pipe, water pipe (also called a *bong*), or rolled into a joint. *Hashish* is a resin made from a concentrate of the flowering tops of the female marijuana plants. Then it is smoked. *Kief* (*kef* meaning "wellbeing" or "pleasure" in Arabic), a similar form of hashish, contains a much higher concentration of psychoactive cannabinoids.

The effect of smoking cannabis is instantaneous but of short duration. They can last for one and a half to four hours. Of course, it will depend on the individual and the cannabinoid concentration of the strain being used.

There is an ongoing debate concerning the link between marijuana smoking and lung cancer. After reviewing nineteen studies, carried out between 1966 and 2006, scientists concluded that there was no statistically significant proof of a correlation between marijuana smoking and lung cancer. On the other hand, the State of California listed cannabis smoke as a cancer agent in 2009. In 2012, the British Lung Foundation concluded, based on literature survey, that cannabis smoke had the potential to produce cancer. Some studies on marijuana smoke have proved the development of pre-cancerous changes of the lung mucous membrane. Cannabis and tobacco smoke are very similar in their compositions. Both contain comparable carcinogen substances.

There is definitely room to take all these studies into account when choosing a delivery method, although smoking cannabis is not associated with the same level of risk than smoking tobacco. Other possible health consequences observed in research carried out to determine the pathological effects of smoked marijuana are airflow obstruction and chronic bronchitis. Emphysema has not been frequently observed.

When smoking, a combustion takes place. According to some sources, the temperature in a joint can reach 2,000 °F (1,093 °C). In contrast, vaporized cannabis (vaping) reaches about 340 °F (171 °C). Therefore, vaporizing is a much more benign delivery method than smoking, and preferred by many marijuana users.

In order to vaporize marijuana, it is necessary to use a special device for this purpose called a *vaporizer*. This process will release cannabinoids. When using a vaporizer, the need to inhale smoke is considerably reduced, and cannabinoids are inhaled without the burning sensation experienced when cannabis is smoked, and without the smell. Some even estimate that the effect of vaporized marijuana is markedly more intense.

The downside of using vaporized cannabis is the cost of the device, which tends to be much more expensive than what is needed to smoke the herb. The quality of vaporizers varies throughout a very wide range. Purchasing a cheap one can produce mediocre results. Therefore, it is wise to do the homework in order to buy one that will fulfill its purpose.

Ingestion

Consuming cannabis orally is an alternative to smoking. When produced for oral consumption, cannabis needs to be infused in oil or butter in order to extract its active substances. The public is misinformed about this delivery method, and therefore it is hard for people to make a decision about whether to use cannabis in edible form or not. It is important to keep certain points in mind in order to benefit as much as possible from using this delivery method. As cannabinoids are metabolized in a different way when they are administered through edibles, the effects are not comparable than when cannabis is smoked or vaporized.

The first thing to have in mind is that edibles can be much stronger than smoked or vaporized cannabis. The variation in potency is also something to point out as their strength depends on the way they are made. When edibles are purchased, it is necessary to read the label in order to get an idea of the potency of the product. When made at home, the smartest thing is to start with a small amount (5 mg) and increase it as one becomes more experienced. Even experienced marijuana smokers can feel overwhelmed if they overdo the amount of edible cannabis they consume, especially if they do so in a short time. The fact that some people have developed a certain degree of tolerance to cannabis through smoked or vaporized marijuana does not necessarily mean that they will tolerate edibles the same way. This type of cross-tolerance is not always present. So we need to be cautious when choosing this delivery method.

Through smoking and vaporization, the time necessary to feel the effects of cannabis is extremely short. In contrast, edible marijuana can take from twenty minutes to one hour (or more) to have an effect. Therefore, we should keep in mind that reaching for more edibles after twenty minutes can bring the person to ingest overwhelming amounts of cannabinoids. That being said, it is recommended to give it at least 45 minutes to one hour before eating more. Some experts even suggest waiting up to two hours in case the person has never had edible cannabis or has not have it for a long time.

As mentioned before, consumption of cannabis in edible form has a different metabolism than when smoked or vaporized. THC is metabolized in the liver into a compound called 11-hydroxy-THC that crosses the *hematoencephalic barrier* very efficiently and is 5-10 times stronger than the THC originally ingested. Edible cannabis has a much longer lasting effects.

It should be clear that edibles have a different effect depending on the person, even more than when cannabis is smoked or vaporized. This difference is rooted in the different way each person digests and metabolizes nutrients. Also our digestive systems work differently depending on certain external and internal conditions, so edibles may not work exactly the same way if we compare their effects when they are ingested in different days. Consequently, we need caution in order to have a positive experience when ingesting edibles.

Some patients use edible cannabis one hour before going to sleep to help them deal with sleep disturbances. This practice could possibly help people with certain degrees of addiction to benzodiazepines in their effort to decrease their withdrawal syndrome. Further discussion is needed in order to confirm this point.

In any case, when choosing edibles as a delivery method, the dose has to be increased gradually and wait to analyze the effects. Using edibles on an empty stomach will intensify their effect. In case too much edibles are ingested, and their effects are felt too intensely, it is important to relax and wait until they wear off. Edible cannabis does not cause long-term toxicity. It is important to stay hydrated once the effects start to be felt, which can last between four and six hours.

Transdermal Administration

Topical medicinal cannabis is another known delivery method, but THC used in this form is not psychoactive. Where marijuana is legal for medicinal purposes, different products are available in the market. These products can be applied topically and include creams, balms and lotions, among other preparations. Anecdotal evidence shows that topical cannabis can be used effectively for conditions like psoriasis, migraines, rheumatoid arthritis, and muscle soreness. The effect of this transdermal delivery method is only local.

Sublingual Administration

Tinctures, which are preparations of concentrated medical cannabis in alcohol, can be used sublingually or mixed with other drinkable liquids. The effects of using this delivery method can be felt within a range of 15 minutes to one hour. It is recommended to start with low doses (5 mg) as with edible cannabis products.

Part 7: Mental Health and Cannabis

Cannabis for Treatment of PTSD

Post-traumatic stress disorder (PTSD) is a serious problem in the modern world. From soldiers returning from war to survivors of workplace shootings and sexual assault, men and women around the world are struggling to put violence behind them and move on with their lives.

Although PTSD has been a recognized disorder for decades now, scientists and doctors still have few options for treating it effectively. *Cognitive therapy* has shown some promise, but the results are still uneven. Some physicians have prescribed *antipsychotic medications* and similar drugs to treat PTSD, but the side effects often cause sufferers to discontinue treatment.

Surprisingly enough, one of the oldest known self-treatments for anxiety and other stress disorders is showing some of the greatest promises. Cannabis has been undergoing serious study to understand the real benefits for men and women suffering from PTSD and related anxiety disorders.

Researchers have long recognized the relationship between marijuana and anxiety, but they often dismissed it as self-medication. For years, scientists thought that people suffering from PTSD turned to marijuana out of desperation, and treatment often focused on getting them to stop taking the drug. Instead of examining the impact cannabis was having on their PTSD, experts assumed that the self-medication was harmful.

All that may be changing as more research into the effectiveness of marijuana in treating PTSD and anxiety comes to light. While the fact that cannabis is still illegal under Federal law makes research difficult, a number of forward-looking scientists have been making real inroads and demonstrating just how well cannabinoids treat PTSD and other anxiety disorders.

The fact that there is currently no specialized effective medication for the treatment of PTSD makes continuing research into the potential effectiveness of cannabis even more critical. PTSD is extremely common among combat veterans. Studies show that as many as 20% of combat vets experience severe PTSD symptoms, including constant stress, nightmares, and flashbacks. Getting those symptoms under control is essential if these brave vets are to live normal lives in the civilian world. Recent studies suggest that marijuana derivatives have a real role to play.

Some studies into the effectiveness of cannabinoids have focused on theses substances interaction in those areas of the brain linked to *emotional memory*, which are severely affected in people displaying signs of PTSD. Research has shown that men and women with PTSD had lower levels of anandamide than did normal volunteers. As we know, anandamide is an endogenous cannabinoid compound, and that may be why cannabis derivatives have shown so much effectiveness in treating the disorder.

Since individuals suffering from PTSD have a deficiency in the endocannabinoid system, bringing that system back into balance can ease the symptoms and help people live more normal lives.

While more research still needs to be done, there is reason to believe that cannabis will play a role in the future treatment of PTSD and other anxiety disorders. As PTSD becomes more and more common, research into effective treatment of the disorder will become increasingly important.

Treating Depression

Depression is a major problem in the modern world. According to the National Institute of Mental Health, almost 9% of young adults suffer at least one episode of major depression, and rates among other age groups are similarly alarming.

With depression accounting for nearly 3% of all new disability claims, governments, health care professionals, and social workers have been searching for a more effective way to treat this serious disease. Current antidepressant medications on the market can have serious drawbacks and potentially dangerous side effects. In fact, some of the most popular medications designed to treat major depression have side effects that include suicidal thoughts.

That may be why so many people who suffer from depression have been looking at alternatives to prescription medication. Cannabinoid compounds have shown great promise in treating depression and anxiety, and research is underway in places where such studies are permitted by law.

A new study reported in the Huffington Post suggests that cannabis could indeed be effective at treating depression, anxiety and related disorders. There has been anecdotal evidence suggesting this linkage for years, but research has been slow in happening due to the legal status of marijuana and its derivatives. Now that a number of states have legalized marijuana for both medical and recreational use, a new age of research is emerging, and the results so far look promising.

The study cited in the Huffington Post article comes from the Research Institute at the University of Buffalo, where neuroscientists found that cannabinoids may be helpful in treating depression that arises as the result of chronic stress.

The studies also found that chronic stress reduced the production of these cannabinoids in the brain. While conducted in rats, the effects in humans may be similar. Endocannabinoids are known to affect cognition, emotion and behavior in a number of different species.

Scientists induced chronic stress in rats through experimental means. Once the rats were properly stressed, the researchers administered cannabinoids from marijuana. The results found that these cannabinoids provided an effective way to restore the natural endocannabinoid levels in the rats' brains. It is thought that the restoration of endocannabinoids may help alleviate some symptoms of depression in human subjects.

Specific strains of cannabis can be particularly valuable in treating depression. One of the most commonly recommended strains of cannabis for depression is known as *Dr. Grinspoon*, after the researcher and Harvard Medical School professor who advocated for cannabis for more than four decades. The Dr. Grinspoon strain belongs to the sativa lineage, and it has also been used to treat nausea in cancer patients.

Other strains of cannabis that are routinely used to treat depression include Hindu Kush, Lemon Kush, Purple Haze, White Rhino and LA Confidential. All of these strains have been used successfully by people suffering from various types of depression and anxiety.

Even though recent studies and anecdotal experience both find promise in cannabinoids for the treatment of depression, researchers urge the public to proceed with caution. The relationship between marijuana usage and depression is a very complicated one, and people should not use the recent studies as an excuse to indulge. Past studies have shown an association between regular marijuana use and depression, and further research is still ongoing. Anyone suffering from depression, anxiety or PTSD should work closely with their doctor to determine the best course of treatment. Self-medication with cannabis or its derivatives is not recommended. As the research into cannabinoids for treating depression continues, new forms of treatment are likely to be developed.

Cannabis and other Psychiatric Disorders

Some people argue that cannabis only serves to make psychiatric disorders such as anxiety, *bipolar disorder*, and schizophrenia worse, while others insist that it is not only harmless, but potentially therapeutic. The truth, however, is much more complex. Though research in this area is often still in its early stages, it has already produced important findings about the role of cannabis in these disorders.

Anxiety

Cannabis has an interesting relationship with anxiety. On the one hand, mild anxiety is a common side-effect that some people report after using cannabis. On the other, there are also many who self-medicate and are even prescribed cannabis to treat a variety of anxiety disorders.

These downright opposite effects that cannabis can have on anxiety may have something to do with the kind of cannabis being used, as well as how different people's bodies react to the chemicals in the plant. For example, strains with high levels of THC might be more likely to produce anxiety, while strains with relatively high levels of CBD often produce a more calming effect.

Bipolar Disorder

Anecdotal evidence suggests that cannabis can lessen the symptoms of bipolar disorder in certain individuals, but several studies have found that the use of cannabis may cause both manic and depressive episodes to increase in severity and frequency. Evidence also suggests that cannabis can trigger bipolar symptoms in susceptible individuals and that it is associated with an earlier onset of the disorder.

However, researchers doubt that cannabis plays a primary causative role in the development of bipolar disorder. Some studies have also shown that marijuana use can improve neurocognitive functioning in bipolar individuals. Patients who use cannabis have displayed better performance on tasks of memory and attention than patients who do not.

Schizophrenia and Psychosis

Studies have demonstrated that cannabis users are more likely to show symptoms of psychosis, and that cannabis use can cause schizophrenia to develop at an earlier age. However, many researchers hypothesize that it is genetics which predispose individuals to both schizophrenia and the desire to use substances such as cannabis. While cannabis may play a role in how and when schizophrenia manifests, one's risk for developing the disorder seems largely to be determined by one's genes.

Furthermore, a number of exciting studies have shown that the CBD compound which is found in the cannabis plant is an effective treatment for psychosis. Better yet, patients report that CBD comes with none of the many unpleasant side-effects of typical antipsychotics.

The Need for More Research

Many mental health practitioners agree that there is therapeutic potential in cannabis, but no consensus has been reached about when and what type of cannabis use may be harmful or helpful for people suffering from anxiety, bipolar disorder, schizophrenia, and psychosis. Certain patients should no doubt steer clear of cannabis, but others may benefit from cannabis use as a form of treatment. More research on the topic would be a great help to both doctors and patients in making important decisions about treatment plans and options.

Cannabis and Sexuality

Scientists have been curious about the effects of cannabis on sexuality for decades, hindered from exhaustive research due to restrictions on the growth and distribution of the plant. Now, though, as more states in America legalize cannabis, the question of whether marijuana enhances or decreases libido for men and women is coming into the foreground. The results of studies to date are a mixed bag, with a definitive answer still very much up for grabs.

In studies such as those by Weller (1984), Hathaway (2003), and Osborne and Fogel (2008), respondents reported that they felt an increase in libido while experiencing the psychoactive effects of cannabis. The percentage of individuals for whom this was true varies, ranging anywhere from one to two-thirds. Conversely, other works, such as the one led by Pitts (2005), indicates that marijuana can cause sexual problems, particularly among men. Looking at more than 8,600 Australians, Pitts found that male cannabis smokers who indulged on a daily basis were four times as likely to experience sexual dysfunction. The same study, however, found that other male respondents suffered from an increase in libido three times as much as those who didn't smoke, and women who smoked experienced problems no more than females who stayed away from the drug.

Some researchers point out that marijuana has a long history of use as an *aphrodisiac* that reaches back hundreds of years. However, the bulk of studies haven't established a firm correlation between marijuana and an increase in libido, although the use of the drug might loosen inhibitions.

Multiple factors could be playing a role in the unpredictable results cannabis seems to produce in regard to libido. For starters, THC and other compounds in cannabis can vary significantly from strain to strain, and how a person consumes or takes in the drug has an influence on how the body reacts. Secondly, as Brown and Dobs (2002) note, even though marijuana can have a suppressive effect on multiple endocrine systems, including those related to reproduction, repeatedly taking the drug may cause users to develop a tolerance. The exact stage of the hormonal cycle a person is in when they use the drug also might affect results. Lastly, cannabis activates brain cell receptors. This can be positive in that it can alter an individual's sense of space, touch and color, but it also can be negative, as nervous system responses can result in elevated heart rate, higher anxiety, paranoia and other issues that decrease libido.

Although evidence suggests that cannabis can lower inhibitions, the relationship between cannabis and libido is less clear. Factors like biology, frequency of use and the exact chemical makeup of a dose may play a role in whether the drug boosts it in certain individuals. People cannot yet take marijuana knowing without a doubt that it will improve this aspect of their lives.

Cannabis-Induced States and Brainwaves

The psychoactive chemicals of the cannabis plant have many different effects on the human body and mind. Arguably, one of the most intriguing effects is the way in which cannabis alters the brain's electrical activity. Known as brainwaves, the pattern of electrical activity in the brain has some interesting correlations with cannabis-induced states.

What Are Brainwaves?

Brainwaves represent the combination of the electrical activity created by the billions of neurons that make up the brain. The frequencies of these brainwaves are grouped into five different types, from lowest to highest frequency, each representing a different mental state.

Gamma waves are the fastest and are usually associated with complex information processing. Beta waves dominate our normal waking consciousness, while alpha waves represent an awake but relaxed and calm state of mind. Theta waves generally emerge when the brain is asleep, or during states of deep meditation or hypnosis when the conscious mind withdraws from the senses. Finally, delta waves represent the slowest frequency and are generally only present in deep, dreamless sleep.

How Does Cannabis Affect Brainwaves?

Using *EEG scans*, researchers have found that cannabis causes brainwaves to slow down. The brain spends the majority of the cannabis high displaying lower alpha and theta frequencies, and, even when not under the influence of cannabis, regular users have been found to generate more powerful alpha waves than non-users. Cannabis use also seems to increase delta waves during sleep. Since dreams usually occur in *REM (Rapid Eye Movement)* sleep and REM sleep is characterized by the faster theta waves, this would explain why cannabis users report having fewer dreams than non-users.

The Paradox of the Cannabis High

If faster brainwaves are associated with higher levels of awareness, then how is it that the cannabis high, which decreases the frequency of brainwaves, creates a subjective experience of heightened perception?

As we know now, higher frequency—or faster—brainwaves are correlated with a more intense mental activity and information processing. The greater use of our executive functions such as working memory, problem-solving, and planning demands from us to retrieve information from the past and forecast what might occur in the future. On the other hand, lower frequency—or slower—brainwaves are associated with and increased subconscious activity and a more passive state of mind in terms of reasoning and other executive functions. Therefore, we tend to focus less on the past and the future and concentrate more on the present. In other words, our expectations and assumptions tend to decrease the further we move away from consciousness and towards a subconscious and passive state of mind.

During the cannabis high, we experience a pronounced focus on the here and now. Our perception of time and the world surrounding us changes. Time seems to slow down and our power to perceive through our senses is enhanced. Although, in such a state of mind, we still retrieve information from the past, our preoccupation with it seems to fade. Cannabis allows us to enter such a level of consciousness that we remain awake while still in touch with our subconsciousness.

As the mental activity associated with faster brainwaves quiets down, it also becomes easier to attend to our inner world. Without all of the assumptions that normally filter their thoughts and ideas, many people develop new insight and understanding into mental or emotional problems. Some even find that the quieter and more relaxed state of mind brought about by the cannabis high is very conducive to creative insights and epiphanies.

The research into cannabis-induced states and brainwaves is still in its infancy, but the intriguing correlations that have been discovered so far provide ample reason to continue. From relaxation to epiphanies, to self-realization, the slower brainwaves associated with cannabis-induced states have many potential benefits.

Part 8: Understanding Addiction

Today, there's a general perception in the public from those with little knowledge about cannabis that marijuana is not addictive. In truth, it is. And it has been proven by serious research like the studies carried out by Anthony in 1994 and López-Quintero in 2011. These studies concluded that roughly 1 in 11 cannabis users become dependent. This rate is higher among those who start consuming cannabis as teenagers (1 in 6) and even higher among heavy users (1-2 in 4). In spite of these findings, we need to understand the problem of addiction in a non-emotional way so we can benefit of the positive properties of the cannabis plant. Also, comparing the addictive potential of cannabis with the addictive potential of other substances will allow us to have a better grasp of the extent of marijuana's dependence risks.

Before elaborating on this subject, I'd like readers to become more familiar with certain concepts that will allow to understand what addiction means. We'll define the following terms: *neurotransmitters, receptors, drug tolerance, dependence* or *addiction*, and the *harm reduction principle*.

Neurotransmitters are biochemical agents that have an inhibitory or excitatory effect when they bind to specific receptors, which are molecules embedded in the cells membrane. To illustrate this concept, we will mention one neurotransmitter found in the central nervous system named *GABA* (gamma-aminobutyric acid), a primary inhibitory neurotransmitter. *Benzodiazepines*, for example, a category of drugs prescribed as anxiolytics and hypnotics (and sometimes as *anticonvulsants*), enhance the effect of GABA. Therefore, these medications help decrease anxiety and have a sleep inducing effect.

Drug tolerance develops when, in order to get the expected effect of the drug, the individual needs to progressively increase the dose of the substance, as its efficacy diminishes with its continuous use. In the case of benzodiazepine tolerance development, GABA progressively loses its inhibitory power. Accordingly, the drug becomes less effective in diminishing anxiety or inducing sleep, and the central nervous system becomes more excitable. In the case of benzodiazepines, all of this can happen within days or weeks.

The development of tolerance can lead to physical dependence or addiction, usually coupled with psychological addiction. Dependence or addiction is characterized by the development of tolerance, *withdrawal symptoms*, and a pattern of behavior marked by the obsessive drive to procure the drug despite the certainty of its destructive effects and the harm that this conduct is causing to the individual, socially and financially.

Harm Reduction: A Sensible Approach

This concept is conceived as an alternative to abstinence and seeks to understand the fact that drugs are used for different purposes, some of them positive. In a sense, harm reduction is the basis of all pharmacological treatments prescribed by physicians who seek to diminish the patient's exposure to risks and, therefore, make a particular treatment or behavior safer. We must not forget that every medication, in whatever form, has some kind of side effect and needs to be administered according to certain criteria and within a safe *therapeutic range*.

Many governments and even health care practitioners take an approach to drugs and addiction that rules out the possibility of substituting a safer drug for a much more dangerous one. This sort of ideologically driven approach to addiction treatment, however, does nothing to help the addicts themselves.

Let's go back to cannabis. All elements that characterize dependence have been found in cannabis users, especially in individuals who are (maybe genetically) predisposed to addiction. According to the National Institute of Drug Abuse (NIDA), about 9% of cannabis users become abusers. As we mentioned, some people are more vulnerable than others, although the potential for addiction is present in everyone.

There is another neurotransmitter whose role is well-known in the study of addiction. It is called *dopamine* and sometimes dubbed "the pleasure hormone." Dependence-producing drugs like *cocaine* and *heroin* flood the brain with dopamine. A structure especially involved in the biochemical function of dopamine is the *nucleus accumbens*, which is a center tied to motivation, pleasure, and reward.

To be sure, there is an addictive potential when abusing cannabis. However, if we compare the risk of becoming dependent through cannabis consumption with the risk of addiction when using other substances, we see that the addictive potential of marijuana is relatively low: cannabis 9%, alcohol 15%, cocaine 17%, opiates 23%, and nicotine 32% (Interestingly, research carried out at Johns Hopkins University in Baltimore showed that 50% of regular coffee drinkers experienced withdrawal symptoms when they didn't have their coffee, and 13% felt sick enough to see their work performance impaired.) In addition, withdrawal symptoms caused by quitting marijuana are not comparable in terms of severity to most other substances of abuse. They are much milder. Let's just take the example of alcohol consumption discontinuation: *delirium tremens* is associated with a 30% risk of death.

Despite its addictive potential, and according to some studies, there are many people who prefer to substitute the use of cannabis for the use of alcohol and other addictive prescription drugs like benzodiazepines. There is a perceived reality that marijuana has fewer undesirable side effects and is marked by fewer negative issues with withdrawal. It seems that, for most people, quitting cannabis is much easier than quitting tobacco or alcohol. Tolerance to cannabis also seems to take longer to set in. It can take months or even years. Whereas with drugs like benzodiazepine, dependence sets in in a matter of a few weeks.

As far as harm reduction is concerned, it is possible to meet people that have managed to find the right cost/benefit balance. They have reached a level where they can optimize the benefits of cannabis consumption and decrease its risks to the minimum. The optimum way to accomplish this is under the supervision of physicians with genuine concern for their patients.

An interesting social phenomenon has been the increase in the number of patients undergoing rehab for marijuana addiction during the last years. According to a study carried out by Copeland and Maxwell in 2007, 69% of the people on treatment for marijuana dependence were coerced by the criminal justice system and went into rehab after been arrested for possession and then put on probation. Consequently, the fact that the number of people going through rehab for "marijuana addiction" has increased may not constitute a measure of the addictive potential of the substance.

Maybe it is time to revisit our paradigm regarding the use of cannabis and our understanding of its addictive power. About 50% of cannabis abusers treated in clinics in the United States have an underlying psychiatric disorder like depression, anxiety, PTSD (post-traumatic stress disorder), and schizophrenia. On the other hand, we see that cannabis can bring a tangible benefit to many people in need of its medicinal properties to deal with their ailments. The harm reduction doctrine could very well be applied to cannabinoids use as well.

Physical Addiction

Addiction is a complex phenomenon caused by the interplay of biology and psychology. Though the biological and psychological components of addiction cannot be entirely disentangled from one another in any given individual, exploring each component separately can contribute to a more complete understanding of addiction as a whole. On a purely physical level, the compulsive and potentially destructive behavior which characterizes addiction is thought to be the result of structural and biochemical changes in the brain.

How Addiction Hijacks the Brain

The brain is made up of cells called neurons, which communicate with one another using chemicals known as neurotransmitters. Different neurotransmitters activate different neuronal receptors, producing the array of perceptions and emotions experienced by the human being.

Feelings of pleasure and reward occur when the neurotransmitter dopamine is released into an area of the brain known as the nucleus accumbens. The brain is designed to be able to handle the mild, intermittent bursts of dopamine which occur naturally in life. Drugs of abuse, however, hijack the brain's natural pleasure and reward pathway, flooding it with high levels of dopamine for a prolonged period of time.

Certain behaviors can stimulate the release of dopamine and cause addiction as well. For example, while nicotine is a physically addicting substance, many smokers find it so difficult to quit because even the hand-to-mouth motions of smoking can produce feelings of pleasure. Internet addiction is also fast becoming an area of concern and has been the topic of much addiction research in the past few years.

The Role of Tolerance in Physical Addiction

Dopamine is one of the brain's most important neurotransmitters. Not only does it play a role in feelings of pleasure and reward, but also in movement, memory, attention, and perception. When levels of dopamine fall out of balance, it can have a devastating impact on an individual's ability to function. Substances and behaviors which stimulate the overproduction of dopamine will eventually cause the development of tolerance, which is essentially the brain's way of protecting itself.

Tolerance is created via a combination of two main biochemical processes, downregulation and desensitization. Downregulation occurs when the brain both eliminates dopamine receptors and produces less dopamine. Desensitization further serves to make the brain's pleasure pathway less efficient by inactivating many of the dopamine receptors which remain.

On a subjective level, the mechanisms of downregulation and desensitization create a numbed pleasure response. The addict finds that the substance or activity they used to derive pleasure from has become less pleasurable. They must now seek out even more of the substance or activity in order to achieve the same effect.

The Role of Dependence in Physical Addiction

High tolerance can prompt an addict to increase their drug-taking activity to the point that the brain begins to depend on the drug. This is where drug addiction and behavioral addictions diverge. Both types of addictions can hijack the brain's reward circuitry and result in desensitization. Addictive behaviors, however, are not generally capable of causing outright physical dependence because they do not involve the introduction of an external substance into the body.

Once the brain becomes physically dependent on a drug, the addict rarely experiences the same high that they used to feel upon using it. Rather, the brain adapts in such a way that the substance becomes incorporated into its regular biochemical functioning. The drug is now not only tolerated, but required to maintain normal cell function.

The terms "dependence" and "addiction" are often used interchangeably, but it is worthwhile to note that "dependence" describes the brain's physical need for a substance while "addiction" refers to the uncontrollable cravings and self-destructive behaviors of the addict. The two do usually go hand-in-hand, but not in every situation.

Withdrawal and Physical Addiction

An addict will experience withdrawal if they go too long without using the substance that their brain has become dependent on. Many people initially begin using drugs for the high and the pleasurable effects, but, once they become dependent, the goal of drug-seeking behavior turns from the attainment of pleasure to the prevention of pain.

Because the brain has incorporated the substance into its regular biochemical functioning, withdrawal is usually characterized by effects opposite of those produced by the drug. If the brain learns to rely on a drug to carry out certain functions, then it will no longer be able to carry out those functions on its own. Different drugs can produce different withdrawal symptoms for this reason.

However, what researchers have called "withdrawal syndrome" is often marked by similar symptoms regardless of which specific substance one is addicted to, mainly because of dopamine depletion. Mild symptoms of withdrawal include tremors, sweating, headaches, irritability, increased heart rate, and nausea. Prolonged and heavy substance abuse can lead to more serious symptoms of withdrawal such as depression, anxiety, confusion, seizures, and even hallucinations.

Can Physical Addiction Be Treated?

A physical addiction often wreaks havoc on a person's life, especially if left untreated. The biochemical and structural brain changes caused by tolerance and dependence make it incredibly difficult to kick an addiction on one's own. A period of detoxification is usually needed in order to begin the treatment process, followed by medication to help one manage the symptoms of withdrawal.

Therapy is also a very important tool for both the treatment of addiction and the prevention of relapse. A person who is no longer addicted to a certain substance or behavior may nevertheless still have the same psychological or social triggers that led them to addiction in the first place. If these problems are not addressed and properly dealt with, then they may return to their old habits and fall into a physical addiction once again.

Brain and Behavior

Physical addiction provides a powerful example of how behavior can impact the brain, and of how the brain, in turn, can impact behavior. Someone's initial choice to do addictive drugs or continually seek out a pleasurable activity results in physical and measurable brain changes, which then causes the need for more of the same behavior. Addiction is a cycle which fuels itself, and the more we understand that cycle, the better equipped we may become to break it.

Psychological Addiction

What is it that determines how likely someone is to become dependent on or completely addicted to a certain substance or behavior? One part of the answer, particularly when the substance in question produces withdrawal symptoms, is a biological one. Some people become hooked because their body begins to need that substance in order to function properly. Addiction, however, is possible even when a substance does not cause any physical addiction in the body, and even physical addiction usually comes with a strong psychological component.

Psychological addiction is often not as well understood or taken as seriously as physical addiction. However, a psychological addiction can be just as debilitating as a physical one. Some people may even find it harder to kick a mental craving long after a physical one is gone. Psychological addiction is often rooted in an individual's most powerful emotions, wants, needs, and desires, and understanding it is crucial to understanding addiction as a whole.

Negative Emotions and Psychological Addiction

One of the main reasons that people become psychologically addicted to certain substances and behaviors is because they are trying to mask or distract themselves from strong negative feelings such as depression and anxiety. In this case, the addict is essentially self-medicating their unpleasant emotional state. Alcohol addiction is a classic example of the role that negative emotions play in psychological addiction. While prolonged use does create a strong physical dependence, many people first turn to alcohol because it offers them a reprieve from feeling anxious or depressed.

The reprieve afforded by turning to substances or behaviors in order to relieve psychological discomfort is, of course, always temporary. When the relief wears off and the negative feelings come back, some people find themselves turning to the substance or behavior again. This creates a relentless cycle that leads to addiction. The cycle is often exacerbated even further when, because they haven't been dealt with them in a psychologically healthy way, the negative emotions come back even stronger than before.

But how do we account for the fact that some people dealing with anxiety and depression become addicts while others do not? Researchers speculate that the likely determining factor is something known as effortful control. Defined as the ability to control one's emotions and impulses, effortful control can impact addiction in two ways.

Firstly, having low levels of effortful control can make it harder for someone to shift their attention away from their negative emotions, increasing the need to search for an immediate form of distraction. Secondly, once the distraction has been found in the form of a substance or a behavior, an individual with low levels of effortful control will find it more difficult to stop.

Positive Emotions and Psychological Addiction

While some people turn to substance abuse or unhealthy behavior because of overwhelming negative emotions, others can get caught in the cycle of addiction because of an increased sensitivity to positive emotions. Simply put, because a certain substance or behavior gives them pleasure, they seek to repeat it again and again. This can result in both a strong psychological need for the behavior or substance, and, if their chosen substance is physically addictive, it can also lead to a physical addiction in the body.

Positive emotional states have also been extensively linked in the psychological research to risk-taking behavior. It seems that individuals who feel positive emotions more often and more intensely are increasingly likely to, for example, try a potentially addictive substance in the first place. This personality trait, often dubbed "positive urgency," has been found to be especially prevalent among college-aged students who develop drug and alcohol problems.

Effortful control also plays an important role in psychological addiction stemming from positive emotions. Many people are able to feel intense and heightened pleasure, but not all struggle with addiction. Addiction is most likely to impact those who are unable to distract themselves from their positive emotions and who therefore find it more difficult to ignore their impulses.

Addiction and a Search for Purpose

Though many people's psychological addictions stem from the positive or negative affective states described above, others may develop one because of a general lack of emotional investment in life.

Some individuals fall into addiction out of a need to fill an inner sense of emptiness.

Addictive behaviors and substances can provide these individuals with a means of escape from a life that they see as meaningless and without purpose, and can even come to be seen as a sort of purpose in and of themselves. For example, while cannabis does not usually produce a strong physical addiction in most users, some people can become dependent on using it to change their ordinary consciousness and experience of the world.

Social isolation and boredom can also contribute to the development of a psychological addiction, especially in people on the fringes of society. Some individuals who find themselves homeless and jobless end up turning to drugs just for something to do to pass the time, and as a means of distracting themselves from their current situation. This can be difficult to understand for people who can simply flick on the TV, turn on the computer, or open a book whenever boredom hits.

Furthermore, without a network of social support, at-risk individuals likely don't have anyone around to catch the signs of a developing addiction, nor any real motivation to seek treatment even if they recognize their own problem. Having strong and meaningful social connections is one of the most important components of keeping people from falling into an addiction, and of getting them out of one.

Addiction and the Individual

As you can see, emotions, wants, needs, and deep-seated desires play an incredibly important role in determining what sorts of substances and behaviors someone might become addicted to, and even how susceptible they are to developing an addiction in the first place. Though these intangible mental phenomena can't be measured in a lab, they can nevertheless have a very real and undeniable effect on human behavior.

Hypersensitivity and Addiction

Hypersensitivity has become an increasingly popular buzzword in the fields of psychology and neurology over the past several years. Researchers have also recently started taking a look at how the hypersensitive personality trait contributes to the development and progression of addiction.

This is an intriguing area of study because of what it can show us about how and why addiction affects different people differently. Before delving into the intricacies of how hypersensitivity and addiction interact, however, it will be beneficial to gain a good understanding of hypersensitivity itself.

What is Hypersensitivity?

Hypersensitivity is a personality trait exhibited by about 20% of the population in equal numbers of men and women. Commonly known in the scientific literature as highly sensitive persons (HSPs), these individuals' experience of the world differs in some important ways from the experience of non-HSPs.

HSPs display a greater depth of processing for both sensory and emotional stimuli, greater sensitivity to subtle stimuli, and higher levels of physiological arousal than the general population. Studies have found that HSPs show greater brain activation of high-order visual processing areas when exposed to visual stimuli, as well as more activation in regions associated with empathy when looking at the faces of loved ones.

Because of their heightened sensory processing, HSPs are often more easily overwhelmed by both emotional and physical stress. They tend not to like overly loud or bright environments, and have a propensity for taking on the negative emotions of others as their own. Hypersensitivity, however, should not be viewed as a wholly negative personality trait. Because they have the ability to process so much sensory information at once, HSPs are often very astute and attentive to detail. They also report having an extremely rich and multi-faceted inner life which often manifests itself in creativity and inventiveness.

As with all personality traits, the way that hypersensitivity interacts with one's environment and upbringing is a crucial part of determining how it will ultimately impact one's life.

How Hypersensitivity May Lead to Addiction

In a 2006 paper titled "The Clinical Implications of Jung's Concept of Sensitiveness (Elaine N. Aron)," it explains that HSPs who experienced trauma in childhood were later more prone to developing symptoms of depression and anxiety than non-HSPs with similar experiences. Furthermore, the authors of a 2008 study titled "Sensory-processing sensitivity in social anxiety disorder: Relationship to harm avoidance and diagnostic subtypes (Hoffman and Bitran)" found that hypersensitivity was strongly associated with generalized social anxiety disorder. Individuals with hypersensitivity were more likely to go out of their way to avoid social situations and public spaces due to the anxiety it caused them.

It is well known in addiction research that mood disorders are strongly linked to addiction. People with anxiety and depression sometimes turn to drugs or alcohol as a way of self-medicating and finding relief from negative emotions. It seems that, when an individual's environment and upbringing aren't conducive to developing the benefits of being highly sensitive, an HSP may turn to substance abuse in order to cope with the resulting emotional problems. HSPs, because they experience emotions so intensely, may find it even more difficult than non-HSPs to successfully distract themselves from their negative emotions on their own, making drugs or alcohol an even more appealing solution.

HSPs may also face a heightened risk of addiction because of a combination of genetic and biochemical factors. Published in 2009, a paper titled "Beyond Diathesis Stress: Differential Susceptibility to Environmental Influences (Belsky and Pluess)" revealed just how powerful of an effect genes could have on personality traits and susceptibility to addiction. Researchers in this study found that hypersensitivity was strongly associated with the presence of a gene which also resulted in less efficient dopamine receptors in the brain.

Dopamine is implicated in the development of addiction more so than any other neurotransmitter because it is largely responsible for stimulating the brain's pleasure/reward pathway. When the brain has normal levels of dopamine, it is able to derive pleasure from everyday activities such as getting a job well done, engrossing oneself in a stimulating activity, or having a positive social interaction. However, because HSPs may have naturally lower levels of dopamine, they may seek more frequent dopamine-releasing stimulation in order to feel the same sense of reward that a non-HSP would feel.

Furthermore, the same genes associated with lower dopamine levels have also been associated with high novelty seeking behavior, making HSPs more likely to try different methods of stimulating their reward pathways. This can lead HSPs not only to try addictive drugs, but also to over-engage in a variety of other behaviors which can ultimately lead to addiction. It is possible and not at all uncommon to develop addictions to food, sex, online browsing, watching TV, computer games, risky behaviors, and even to relationships.

Any activity in which an HSP can engross themselves in and release dopamine with is susceptible to turning it into an addiction. If the activity no longer produces the same feeling of reward, then it will need to be repeated more often and with greater intensity. For example, someone who has grown to rely on food as a way of releasing dopamine may develop a binge-eating disorder, while someone whose reward pathway has been over-stimulated by Internet browsing may experience symptoms of withdrawal when away from the screen.

Improving Treatment Options for HSPs

Though the studies which have so far been done on different aspects of hypersensitivity have helped to shed some light on how addiction can impact HSPs, there is a glaring need for more robust and focused research on the subject. Gaining an even better understanding of how the unique genetic makeup of HSPs can contribute to their susceptibility to addiction would be an invaluable tool for improving treatment options and prevention strategies.

HSPs have made numerous contributions to society. Many of our best scientists, writers, musicians, artists, teachers, thinkers, and philosophers have no doubt fallen into the HSP category. The more that educators and medical professionals become aware of the unique needs of hypersensitive individuals all the way from childhood to adulthood, the more they can help ensure that society doesn't lose their gifts and talents to addiction.

Dissociation

Dissociation is a term used to describe a state of mind which is characterized by a detachment from one's immediate surroundings or from certain past experiences. It occurs when the normally integrated processes of awareness, perception, memory, and personal identity become disconnected in some way. Dissociative states are highly variable and fall on a continuum from mild to severe or, in other words, from nonpathological to pathological.

Almost everyone has experienced nonpathological states of dissociation in their lives. In fact, most people experience them just about every day. Daydreaming and "zoning out" from the world around you by becoming lost in your thoughts is a mild form of dissociation. Dissociation can also be an effective coping mechanism, and is often used to deal with stress, conflict, and even boredom.

Pathological dissociation, on the other hand, is maladaptive and causes a significant negative impact on how an individual relates to the world. It can include symptoms such as amnesia, derealization, depersonalization, confusion over one's identity, and sometimes even the assumption of a new identity. Depression and anxiety are also commonly associated with dissociative disorders.

Dissociation and Substance Abuse

Some people who suffer from dissociative disorders turn to drugs and alcohol as a way of dealing with the stress, depression, and anxiety caused by their condition. They may find that a certain substance helps to drown out these negative emotions, and so they use that substance more frequently and more copiously in an effort to keep masking their feelings. This eventually leads to tolerance, and then to withdrawal once the substance is taken away, prompting the user to take more.

Another important factor to consider when it comes to the connection between dissociation and substance abuse is that pathological dissociation is often the result of trauma. While many people who have suffered trauma in the form of psychological, physical, and sexual abuse do not go on to develop a dissociative disorder, people with dissociative disorders are more likely to have experienced such abuse than the general population. Researchers have discovered a strong correlation between addiction, dissociation, and early childhood trauma in particular.

A 2013 paper titled "Relationships of Dissociative Disorders and Personality Traits in Opium Addicts on Methadone Treatment" (Ghafarinezhad, Rajabizadeh, and Shahriari) found that dissociative traits as a result of past trauma were more common in people who had developed an opium addiction than in the control group of non-addicts. These findings were corroborated in a 2014 study called "Predicting Addiction Potential on the Basis of Early Traumatic Events, Dissociative Experiences, and Suicide Ideation" (Sajadi et al.), where the authors concluded that addiction potential can be predicted by "early trauma, dissociative experience, and suicide ideation."

Dissociative Drugs
The experience of dissociation is induced naturally by the brain's own neurochemistry, and so it should come as no

surprise that it can also be induced by consuming certain psychoactive substances. Naturally occurring dissociative states can be mimicked by a class of hallucinogens known as dissociatives. Most dissociatives were originally created for medical use but, like numerous other drugs, have come to be used recreationally as well.

The most commonly used dissociative substances are ketamine, phencyclidine (PCP), and dextromethorphan (DXM). PCP and ketamine were both developed for use as surgical anesthetics, while DXM is an active ingredient in many over-the-counter cough suppressants. There are some differences in the effects of these drugs, but all three produce the same general sense of dissociation and detachment from the immediate environment.

At lower doses dissociative drugs can create distortions in one's visual and auditory perceptions. Users often feel as if they are "floating" and may even experience a mild sense of euphoria. At higher doses the effects become even more pronounced and result in dream-like trances and hallucinations, as well as numbness, body tremors, and an impaired ability to move. Amnesia, extreme changes in mood and energy levels, and distortions to one's sense of self may also occur with the use of dissociative drugs.

Dissociative Drug Addiction

Just as with any substance, there are many psychological and physical factors that determine if an individual will become addicted to a dissociative drug. Some people are more likely to develop an addiction if they turn to the use of dissociative drugs as a way of self-medicating psychological problems such as depression, anxiety, and trauma. Dissociatives can seem like an appealing option because they can help one forget their stresses and worries, if only temporarily. The problem is that the feelings come back when the substance wears off, and are sometimes even worse than they were before.

The cycle of addiction may begin if the drug is then continually sought after and taken again. Not only does the user become psychologically dependent on the drug, but taking a dissociative drug often enough and in high enough doses will eventually begin altering one's brain chemistry and cause a physical addiction in the body as well. Dissociative substances imitate and therefore lower the levels of some of the brain's key neurotransmitters, resulting in intense physical cravings and symptoms of withdrawal.

Published in 2000, an article titled "An Approach to Drug Abuse, Intoxication and Withdrawal" (Giannini) discussed how six different classes of drugs affect five neurotransmitters, including dopamine, which play a role in the brain's pleasure and reward circuitry. Only dissociatives, they noted, alter the functioning all five neurotransmitters. The 2015 paper "Introduction: Addiction and Brain Reward and Anti-Reward Pathways" (Gardner) likewise pointed out that dissociatives act on synapses in the nucleus accumbens, a region of the brain that deals with reward, pleasure, motivation, and behavioral reinforcement.

Addiction's Many Starting Points

Some people turn to drugs as a way of coping with their dissociative disorders. Others become hooked on the chemically induced dissociation that occurs after taking dissociative drugs. One group abuses certain substances because they are trying to escape from the stress caused by dissociation, while the other becomes addicted because they are chasing after dissociative states. This complex relationship between dissociation and addiction highlights the fact that addiction often works on a feedback loop that has many different points of initiation.

Comparing Addictive Potentials: Cannabis, Opioids, and Benzodiazepines

A psychoactive drug is a substance which triggers changes in perception and behavior by acting primarily upon an individual's central nervous system. Not all psychoactive drugs, however, affect human beings in the same way. Some are relatively safe and benign, while others result in unhealthy states of dissociation and in dangerous withdrawal symptoms if their use is discontinued.

Cannabis: Addiction and Withdrawal

As we mentioned before, people can find themselves becoming dependent on cannabis, as tolerance to its compounds is built relatively quickly in the body. When both the brain's reward and endocannabinoid systems become overstimulated, the body can begin to crave more cannabis and to produce mild withdrawal symptoms if it isn't able to obtain any.

Some of the most common symptoms of cannabis withdrawal include irritability, restlessness, anxiety, difficulty sleeping, a decrease in appetite, lethargy, mild tremors, and muscle aches. Fortunately, these withdrawal symptoms are often very manageable. Light users generally feel fine after a few days, while heavy users may experience symptoms for a week or two after stopping.

Cannabis Induced Dissociation

Cannabis is generally classified as a hallucinogenic drug, albeit a weak one. While it does produce differences in sensory perception, it rarely produces hallucinations. In fact, cannabis-induced states might better be described as mildly dissociative rather than hallucinatory. The authors of a 2013 study titled "Amygdala activity contributes to the dissociative effect of cannabis on pain perception" (Lee et al.) noted that it was the dissociative effects of cannabis which made it so "remarkably effective" for certain patients who experience "otherwise intractable pain."

It is important to note that the dissociative states often induced by cannabis would not be classed as pathological. The way that cannabis allows users to become detached from their immediate surroundings is similar to the way people naturally daydream or momentarily "check out" from reality. If the ability to check back in remains intact, then these states can actually be beneficial for coping with stress or other negative emotions.

Opioids: Addiction and Withdrawal

Unlike dependence on and withdrawal from cannabis use, addiction to and withdrawal from opioids, often called opioid use disorder, is unarguably worse and much more dangerous. Opioid addiction results in tens of thousands of deaths every year, a number that has unfortunately been climbing over the past few decades.

Symptoms of opioid withdrawal are often severe, forcing addicts to seek out more drugs in an effort to put a stop to the pain and discomfort. Early symptoms of withdrawal after opioid use stops may include sweating, dehydration, anxiety, fatigue, agitation, confusion, and hot and cold flashes. As the withdrawal progresses the addict may experience nausea, vomiting, abdominal cramping, and diarrhea.

Comparing Opioid and Cannabis Dissociations

Dissociation is deemed pathological when it interferes with the way an individual responds to their surroundings and, therefore, causing their behavior to become maladaptive. Pathological dissociation is characterized by amnesia, depersonalization, and derealization. The sufferer may lose a sense of where they are, what they are doing, and even who they are.

Eli Somer, in an essay called "Opioid use disorder and dissociation" (2009), described how the dissociative experiences of opioid drug users bore a similar phenomenology to such pathological dissociative states. He found that the drugs were often used in order to produce a type of

151

"chemical amnesia," as well as "numbing, depersonalization, and derealization."

The nonpathological dissociative states produced by cannabis often help users cope with negative emotions. The pathological dissociative states produced by opioids, on the other hand, can, and frequently do, contribute to even greater feelings of depression and anxiety once the initial high wears off.

Benzodiazepines: Dissociative Effects, Addiction, and Withdrawal

Benzodiazepines are an interesting class of dissociative drug which perhaps aren't as dangerous as opioids, but which can cause severe withdrawal symptoms and should be treated with caution. Benzodiazepines are popularly used to treat conditions such as seizures, insomnia, anxiety, and muscle spasms because of their muscle relaxant and sedative properties.

Short-term use of benzodiazepines doesn't seem to pose much significant risk to patients. However, the main issue with these psychoactive drugs is how quickly patients build tolerance to them. In order for the benzodiazepines to remain effective, then, patients have to increase their dosage and may even end up taking more than one type of benzodiazepine at a time.

Prolonged use of benzodiazepines, especially at high doses, can cause an individual to develop a dependence on the drug. Their body craves more and more and goes into withdrawal when supply is limited or cut off. Withdrawal symptoms from benzodiazepines often include tremors, insomnia, agitation, anxiety, headaches, heart palpitations, nausea, and even panic attacks.

More severe withdrawal symptoms can generally be avoided if dosage is decreased safely and gradually, but a substantial minority of people experience a protracted withdrawal period that can last for many months afterwards.

Cannabis:
Could it Help to Treat Hard Drug Addictions?

Might it be possible to treat addictions to drugs such as opioids and benzodiazepines with cannabis? If it is possible to treat addiction to opioids and benzodiazepines by replacing their use with cannabis, then it should be pursued as an alternative to conventional rehab treatment. Cannabis has the ability to provide the same beneficial effects as other drugs without the dangerous side-effects, to lessen the withdrawal symptoms of harder drugs, and to lessen the need and cravings for harder drugs.

If these ideas are vigorously pursued and carefully studied, then using cannabis to treat hard-drug addictions could save many more lives in the future. It may not be the right choice for everyone, but neither is conventional rehab the right choice for all addicts. The best course of action for society is to have many potential options for people struggling with addiction, and cannabis should definitely be one of them.

While a person is suffering from a protracted benzodiazepines withdrawal syndrome or trying to cope with withdrawal from opioid drugs, some reserachers suggest that perhaps cannabis could help their symptoms and cravings. At least some intriguing research seems to suggest that it could. For example, a 2009 study published in *Neuropsychopharmacology* found that administering THC to rats that were vulnerable to opioid dependence suppressed their sensitivity to morphine and decreased their self-administration of the drug (Morel, Grios, and Dauege).

Similar results have been seen in humans as well. The 2003 study "Cannabis Reduces Opioid Dose in the Treatment of Chronic Non-Cancer Pain" took a look at how, as the title suggests, cannabis was able to significantly reduce dependence on opioids in a small sample of patients with chronic pain (Lynch and Clark). Another interesting study from 2011, published in the *American Journal of Hospice & Palliative Medicine*, concluded that cannabis is a much safer alternative than opioids in palliative care, and opined that it should not be classified as a Schedule I drug (Carter et al.). The study also pointed out that Dronabinol, a 100% THC prescription drug, is classified more lightly under Schedule III.

The fact that cannabis has the potential to help many people can be further solidified by a series of large-scale studies. The first, a 2007 article out of the *Harm Reduction Journal*, explored the question of whether long-term cannabis users who were seeking access to medical marijuana had higher incidences of using other drugs (O'Connell and Bou-Matar). The authors discovered that, rather than acting as a "gateway drug," cannabis may have been "protective" against more harmful agents.

These findings were further corroborated in a 2009 study titled "Cannabis as a substitute for alcohol and other drugs," which examined the alcohol and drug-taking habits of approved medical cannabis users (Reiman). Once again it was found that cannabis was being used by patients as an effective substitute for alcohol and for more harmful illegal and prescription drugs.

Finally, perhaps the most promising findings in support of the idea that cannabis could be used to offset the harm caused by harder drugs were published in a longitudinal 2014 study called "Medical Cannabis Laws and Opioid Analgesic Overdose Mortality in the United States, 1999-2010" (Bachhuber et al.). Researchers in this groundbreaking study concluded that opioid overdose mortality rates were "significantly lower" during their research period in states that had medical cannabis laws than in states that didn't.

When considering the use of cannabis to treat addiction to other dissociative drugs specifically, it seems worthwhile to suggest that indica-dominant strains may be a better choice than sativa-dominant strains. Indica strains more closely mirror the sedative and relaxing properties of strongly dissociative drugs, and would therefore likely decrease both psychological and physical cravings for those drugs. While research in this area is lacking, it would no doubt be a fruitful avenue of study.

Conclusion

We need a new point of reference to deal with cannabis. Despite the negative image built around marijuana, what this plant is and what it can do can't be changed or denied, and the world is progressively becoming aware of its medicinal properties. Everything in the Universe can be considered morally neutral. The purpose we give to something is what makes it good or bad. And in order to use something like cannabis for the right intent, it needs to be regulated. We need rules and bounds so we can use it for our benefit and not to hurt us. And that is the purpose of a legal system that, allowing society to use all the necessary tools for it to grow, regulates the use of those tools so they can be used safely. Cannabis, without proper guidance and supervision, is like any power left without restraint for anyone to use.

In his book *The Structure of Scientific Revolutions*, Thomas Kuhn writes about the concept of "paradigm shift." This idiom has become part of the English language and describes a switch in the way we look at things. Although we can be looking at the same object, a change of lens can allow us to perceive the object from a different perspective. This is what it's needed concerning cannabis today.

In order to change the way we see cannabis, we need to mature as a society. We must start functioning from a higher level of thinking and abandon the old paradigm. There is nothing intrinsically evil in marijuana, as there is nothing inherently bad with alcohol, or even with drugs with hallucinogenic properties. Indeed, many studies have been carried out to show how certain Schedule I hallucinogens can be successfully used to treat hardwired psychological problems under proper professional supervision. Cannabis deserves a new outlook. To deny the use of medical cannabis to patients who are not responsive to epilepsy medication is short-sighted and inconsiderate, to say the least. Not to allow cancer patients to use it in order to ease the side effects of chemotherapy or to patients suffering from unbearable neuropathic pain is outright insensitive.

Nonetheless, the use of cannabis in a way that is not regulated with responsibility can also become a tool of self-destruction. Proofs of marijuana as a gateway substance haven't been conclusive. But this thesis hasn't been absolutely disproved either. So we need to act with caution should we decide to give cannabis a chance. The best harm reduction tool is to seek physicians with experience in the use of cannabis as a medicinal substance and who truly care about their patients.

Medicine is largely connected with money in today's world --much more than it used to be in the past. But there are still doctors that have an honest concern for their patient's health improvement and special effort has to be made in choosing the right one through recommendations or any other means available. This book has been dedicated to people who don't give up and don't feel sorry for themselves, but carry on looking for a solution to their health problems. They will find it if they look hard enough and are willing to leave their comfort zones and look at the problem from a higher level of thought.

Appendices

Appendix 1: How to Make Cannabutter

Marijuana edibles are sought out by many marijuana users as an alternative to smoking or vaporizing, as well as for their unique and longer-lasting effects. Cannabutter is the key to making a whole range of potent and tasty marijuana edibles, and it is easy to make too. All you need is a few simple ingredients and a free afternoon.

Step 1 - Gather your ingredients and supplies. Before starting up your stove, make sure that you have the following ingredients and supplies on hand: finely ground marijuana, butter, a large saucepan, a strainer or cheesecloth, and Tupperware containers.

As a good rule of thumb, you should use about 1 lb. of butter for every ounce of marijuana. If you don't need to make this much cannabutter, then lower the amounts as needed, just make sure you keep the correct ratio.

Step 2 - Bring water to a boil. Put a few cups of water into your saucepan and heat until it is boiling. It doesn't really matter how much water you use, just make sure it will be enough to hold all of the marijuana.

Step 3 - Add butter. Once the water is boiling, reduce it to a medium to low heat setting and add in the butter. Make sure that the butter melts completely, and lower the heat some more if it ever begins burning.

Step 4 - Add the marijuana and simmer. Now you can add the marijuana into your water and melted butter mixture. Keep your mixture on a low heat so that it is just simmering, stirring occasionally. You are going to need to keep simmering for at least 2 to 3 hours. You'll be able to tell when it's ready because the consistency will become thicker, and the top of your mixture will look glossy.

Step 5 - Strain and store overnight. Once your mixture is ready, you need to strain it into a Tupperware container. You can use a regular strainer, but a cheesecloth will probably be easier to use, and it will keep more marijuana out of the final product. Seal the container up and put it in the fridge overnight.

Step 6 - Separate the butter from the water. When you look at your mixture the next day, you'll notice that the butter has separated itself from the water and is sitting on top. Just pour out the wastewater and you should have a nice, green stick of cannabutter that you can now substitute in for the butter in any of your favorite recipes!

Some Tips on Dosing

Marijuana edibles produce a long-lasting, intense high, and it can be easy to get carried away and eat too much. If you used a whole ounce to make cannabutter and then proceeded to use the butter to whip up a batch of brownies, then you don't want to eat all of the brownies at once. Try a few bites at first and give it some time to see how you feel before having more.

Appendix 2: How to Prepare and Use Cannabis Tincture

Tinctures are a whole-plant cannabis alcohol extraction that can be an appealing option for medical cannabis patients because they allow for consistent and controlled dosing. They also offer a fantastic middle ground between smoking/vaporizing and edibles in terms of onset and duration.

Here's how you can do it at home.

Materials and Preparation

Cannabis tinctures are simple to make and don't require many materials. All you'll need is:

- A bottle of 190-proof grain alcohol

- Any amount of vaporized or unvaporized cannabis

- Cheesecloth

- A funnel

- Mason jars

- Aluminum foil and a baking sheet (if using unvaporized cannabis)

- Tinted dropper bottles

Cannabis tincture can be made using vaporized or unvaporized bud. If using unvaporized bud, the cannabis first has to undergo a process known as decarboxylation. This can be done by grinding up your bud, spreading it over a baking sheet, sealing it tightly with foil, and baking it for 45 minutes at 220°F.

If you plan to use cannabis that has been vaporized, then you can skip this step, as it has already been decarboxylated by the vaporizer. Now, whether you used vaped bud or not, the next three steps will be the same:

1) Place the cannabis inside a mason jar and pour enough grain alcohol into the jar to just submerge all of the bud. Tightly seal the jar when you are done.

2) Keep the jar in a cool, dark place for 4 days, giving it a gentle shake a couple of times a day.

3) After 4 days, strain the mixture through a cheesecloth into a large enough

container or cup, then through a funnel into the dropper bottles.

Use and Dosing

Cannabis tincture is usually taken by placing a few drops under the tongue. Even if you are an experienced user, you should start small to see how it affects you. Try two drops at first and wait to see how you feel before taking more. The effects can be felt within around 20 minutes to half an hour, and can last for 2 to 4 hours.

Because the taste isn't very pleasant, some people choose to mix their tincture with a drink. In this case, however, the tincture will be absorbed through your gastrointestinal tract rather than through the mouth's arterial blood supply. The onset and duration would then take longer, making the experience more similar to an edible, but still faster.

Cannabis tinctures can be used medicinally for many of the same conditions as smoking, vaporizing, or edibles. They can be particularly useful for conditions that require a quicker onset than edibles and longer duration than smoking or vaporizing, such as headaches, migraines, muscle and joint pain, arthritis, nausea, anxiety, and sleep problems.

Of course, it is always a good idea to talk to your healthcare provider about the pros and cons of different methods of cannabis ingestion before starting on something new. Cannabis tinctures may not be right for everyone, but they can be an additional method for many patients to find the relief they need.

Appendix 3: Dabbing

There is yet another way to prepare cannabis that has been practiced for quite a number of years. It is called *dabbing* and it involves the consumption of THC-rich resins in smoked or edible form. The word dabbing has the meaning of pressing something against a surface; in this case, what is pressed is *HBO (butane hash oil)* against a hot surface. These extracts can have up to 90% of tetrahydrocannabinol rates.

There are some concerns regarding this form of preparation due to its high levels of THC, which could cause psychological harm, according to some studies. Indeed, there have been cases of people that have ended up at the ER due to the consumption of dabs. The higher risk with this method is involved in its preparation due to the use of butane, which is a highly flammable chemical that has caused explosions and severe injuries in people dabbing at home.

Nevertheless, others justify the production of extracts through dabbing arguing that there are patients that need a very high dose of THC to manage certain health issues. For those patients, dabbing would be a viable solution, and, if prepared by experts, safety concerns can be adequately managed. There are other ways to produce the extracts with the use of carbon dioxide or ice-water, which are much safer.

Appendix 4: The Benefits of Vaporization

Cannabis use was at one time nearly synonymous with the act of smoking. While smoking no doubt remains the most popular method of consuming cannabis, many people are looking for safer and more discreet alternatives. Vaporization has quickly become one of the main alternatives to lighting up a joint, a pipe, or a bong, and is now a go-to method for many cannabis users.

Vaporization: A Safer Alternative

Just like cigarette smoke, the smoke from burning cannabis bud is both harsh on the lungs and full of potentially carcinogenic chemicals. Heavy cannabis smokers are often at an increased risk of respiratory conditions such as chronic bronchitis. The link between cannabis smoke and cancer is not clear, with some studies purporting to show a correlation, but other failing to find any evidence. While science needs more time to come to a consensus on the issue, you can bypass any of the potential risks of smoking by using a vaporizer instead.

Vaporizers do not heat cannabis up past the point of combustion, which is about 392°F (200°C). While joints burn at over 2,000°F (1,093°C), vaporizers generally go up to a temperature of 375°F (190°C) or less, which is perfect for releasing the active cannabinoids such as THC and CBD from cannabis in the form of vapor. No smoke is produced in the process, and this substantially reduces the inhalation of lung irritating and potentially cancer-causing substances.

Types of Vaporizers

There are so many different vaporizers available that it can be difficult to decide which one is right for you. However, they can be broken up into three main types:

1. First, there are the desktop vaporizers. The Volcano is generally considered to be hands down the best desktop vaporizer available, but it does come with a hefty $539-$669 price tag (depending on the model). Two great and more budget-friendly alternatives are the herbalAire and the Extreme Q, both retailing at around $200.

2. Portable vaporizers are designed to be used on-the-go, and are therefore smaller and more discrete, but also slightly less efficient. They tend to cost between $100 and $250. Among the most popular and well-reviewed portable vaporizers on the market are the Pax 2, the Vapir NO2, and the Magic Flight Launch Box.

3. Pen vaporizers are the smallest, most discrete, and also the least expensive, usually costing between $50 and $100. However, they are generally designed to be used with cannabis concentrates, and will end up burning instead of vaporizing dry bud. If you are interested in getting a pen vaporizer, then check out the SOURCE Orb V2 or the O-Phos.

Where Can You Buy Vaporizers?
Buying and owning vaporizers is legal in most jurisdictions, as they can be sold as tobacco paraphernalia. They can be purchased online directly from the manufacturer or, more popularly, from sites such as Amazon. You can also find vaporizers on the shelves of just about any head shop. Please note, however, that it is always in your best interest to brush

up on the laws of your specific jurisdiction regarding cannabis/tobacco paraphernalia before ordering a vaporizer online.

Appendix 5: The Cannabis High and Hangover

The cannabis high is incomparable to the high produced by almost any other drug and is, therefore, hard to categorize along conventional lines. Is it a stimulant or depressive? Does it cause euphoria or anxiety? Does it cause a hangover? The truth is that the effects of cannabis vary considerably from person to person and rely on factors such as mindset, setting, and strain.

The Cannabis High

What most users can generally agree on is that cannabis enhances one's subjective experience of the world. A breakdown of the different aspects of the cannabis high can help us understand what this statement means.

Onset and Duration

Smoking or vaporizing cannabis usually produces an immediate high that reaches its peak in about 15 minutes. The high generally lasts for about 1 to 2 hours (depending on how much was used), and can take another couple of hours to wear completely off.

The effects of orally ingested cannabis are much slower, and can take anywhere from half an hour to an hour and a half to manifest. However, they also last a lot longer, and the peak effects can be felt for 3-4 hours before beginning to decline.

Emotions

One of the main reasons that people use cannabis is that it tends to produce positive feelings ranging from a sense of well-being to euphoria. Many people report that it makes them feel more relaxed, happier, and more talkative.

Some users, on the other hand, report feeling mild anxiety that can be exacerbated by negative thoughts. It is recommended that you take careful consideration of your current mindset before using cannabis.

When such consideration is taken, however, cannabis can have a very beneficial effect even on negative emotions. Some people report that it can help with the mourning process, but only as long as it is used as an aid for facing one's emotions rather than as a means of escape.

Concentration

Though the cannabis high may make one more prone to distractions, it is also characterized by periods of intense focus. Many people report using it as a study and reading aid because it allows them to zone in and shut out all external stimuli. Even the famed physicist Carl Sagan championed cannabis for its role in helping him solve complex problems.

It seems that Sativa dominant strains are particularly well-suited to the task of enhancing focus and concentration, with some of the most popular being Harlequin, Ghost Train Haze, and Headband.

Memory

Cannabis seems to have an adverse impact on short-term memory. Several studies have shown that cannabis produces impairments in tests of recall and recognition. These effects on short-term memory, however, are only temporary and have not been found to persist after the cannabis high wears off. Neither have researchers found any links between cannabis use and long-term memory.

One interesting phenomenon to note is that cannabis can enhance memories of distant events. Users sometimes report experiencing vivid imagery and remembering minute details from the past that they thought they had forgotten.

Thinking

Cannabis is commonly used to stimulate introspection and self-reflection. In fact, one of the main differences between cannabis and alcohol intoxication is that thinking during the cannabis high is often reported to be clearer. Many users even experience a great increase in the speed of their thoughts, sometimes to the point of having two or more thoughts at once.

On the other hand, consuming too much cannabis can also cause slightly muddled and confused thinking, and may even lead to an impairment of judgment. It is always prudent to remember that, even if you feel clear-headed, you are under the influence of a psychoactive substance and should steer clear of activities such as driving.

Creativity

The chosen drug of artists, musicians, and writers everywhere, cannabis has long been linked with creativity. Though oftentimes the cannabis high is prone to produce only fits of giggles over silly ideas or absorption into long and involved fantasies, it can also provide the necessary stimulation for new insights and creative epiphanies.

Furthermore, cannabis has a unique way of opening the mind and making one more tolerant and accepting of new ideas. This new perspective on the world often helps people see their problems in a new light and reveals solutions that they may not have considered before.

Perception

The cannabis high produces a significant alteration of conscious perception. Sensations are often described as being more intense. The enjoyment of food and music becomes enhanced. As cannabis is classed as a mild hallucinogenic, some users experience closed-eye visuals or a sense that the world has taken on a "cartoony" quality.

Time seems almost to slow down during the cannabis high as the world takes on a new and deeper significance. You can spend what seems like an hour observing the beautiful woodwork of a coffee table, only to check the time and see that barely five minutes have passed. Cannabis may also produce a slight sense of *depersonalization* or *derealization*, making you feel like an outside observer who is watching your own actions.

The Cannabis Hangover

Though many users swear that it doesn't exist, some people do indeed experience a hangover the day after using cannabis. A cannabis hangover is typically characterized by dry mouth, headache, dry eyes, a sore throat, and a general feeling of grogginess.

Thankfully, these unpleasant side effects can usually be taken care of with a warm shower, moisturizing eye drops, and plenty of water. Most users find that once they can get themselves out of bed and start going about their day, the hangover wears off.

An even better strategy for taking care of the cannabis hangover is to prevent it. If a sore throat is one of your main concerns, then consider vaporizing instead of smoking, or following up a smoke with a soothing drink such as tea. It is also a good idea to sober up before bed or to make sure that you are going to be able to get enough sleep the next morning before lighting up at night. You may even want to consider switching strains. Perhaps you are using a dominant indica strain that is hitting your body too hard.

One of the best things about cannabis is that there are so many options available when it comes to what strain you chose and how you chose to use it. With enough experimentation, you can come to find out which strain, setting, mindset, and method of ingestion works best for you. For example, short-term memory side effects can be offset by using strains with higher rates of cannabidiol, as it was proved in a study published in 2010. In that study, cannabis smokers using strains with high percentages of CBD didn't experience short-term memory issues.

Appendix 6: Suppressing the Appetite-Boosting Effect of Cannabis

It is a well-known phenomenon that consuming cannabis boosts the appetite and often causes users to overeat. Known scientifically as "hyperphagia" and commonly as "the munchies," some people can find this overpowering urge to eat problematic enough to stop using cannabis altogether. The good news is that researchers have discovered many of the reasons behind why cannabis affects the appetite the way that it does, and this information can help us come up with some effective strategies for suppressing the munchies.

How Cannabis Stimulates Appetite

It is important to note that the research on why cannabis stimulates the appetite has so far only been conducted on mice and rats. Nevertheless, scientists use these small rodents because they bear genetic similarities to humans, and discoveries of how mice and rats react to certain conditions often later correlate to how humans are found to react.

The first of these studies was a 2007 paper published in *Neuropsychopharmacology* (Mahler, Smith, and Berridge) which found that cannabis seems to enhance the hedonistic pleasure of eating. These findings were confirmed by another group of researchers in 2012 (De Luca et al.), with the additional discovery that the pleasure chemical dopamine was directly involved in the process.

Not only does cannabis increase the subjective pleasure of eating, it also seems to act directly on the taste buds to enhance sweet taste (Yoshida et al. 2010). Furthermore, because taste and scent are so closely related, it should come as no surprise that, in a 2014 paper published in *Nature Neuroscience*, a team of neuroscientists found that cannabis actually increases sensitivity to smell (Marsicano et al.), essentially triggering feeding by making food smell irresistible.

Aside from acting on the sense organs, researchers have also found that cannabis interacts directly with gut enzymes and sets off a neural mechanism which triggers cravings for fatty foods (DiPatrizio et al. 2011). Generally, in humans as in rats, ingesting fatty foods stimulates the craving for more fatty foods via the body's endocannabinoid system. Cannabis mimics the action of fatty foods in the gut, ramping up fat intake even if you are full.

Finally, a neuronal basis for the munchies was established in a 2015 paper out of the Yale School of Medicine (Koch et al.). In it, researchers discovered that stimulation of certain cannabinoid receptors activated a cluster of hypothalamic pro-opiomelanocortin (POMC) neurons. What's interesting is that POMC neurons are typically responsible for promoting satiety, but cannabis causes them to produce endorphins instead of their usual appetite-suppressant neurochemicals.

Cannabis-Induced Appetite Suppression Strategies

Two of the main reasons why cannabis stimulates the appetite the way it does is that it makes food smell and taste so good that it becomes difficult to resist. It stands to reason, then, that simply removing yourself from a situation where you can smell food, or see it and think about how pleasurable it would be to eat, can help curb your appetite for it. Getting yourself outdoors and distracting yourself with a half hour walk can be a good way to avoid the munchies and do something healthy for your body at the same time.

Of course, taking a walk won't stop cannabis from acting on your neurons and gut enzymes. It may be enough for some people to fight the urge, but, if you tend to experience particularly powerful munchies, then you may need some extra help combating them.

One strategy that cannabis smokers who are also cigarette smokers often utilize is mixing their cannabis with tobacco in the form of a spliff, because the nicotine in tobacco has appetite-suppressant properties that can combat the appetite-stimulating effects of cannabis. The appetite-suppressant effects of nicotine have been extensively studied and confirmed, with a fantastic overview of the literature presented in 2009 paper entitled "Nicotinic Receptor-Mediated Effects on Appetite and Food Intake" (Jo, Talmage, and Role).

There is no universal consensus among smokers on how much tobacco should be used. Many prefer to mix their spliffs 50/50, while others prefer a higher ratio of cannabis or a higher ratio of tobacco. An important note of caution, of course, is that tobacco is harmful to one's health, and so as little as is needed to combat the munchies should be used. If you are not already a cigarette smoker, then it would not be advisable to begin just to combat cannabis-induced appetite.

A good alternative if you are trying to cut down on your tobacco smoking but also seeking a way to suppress your appetite is a smokeless tobacco product known as snuff. When inhaled into the nasal cavity, snuff provides a hit of nicotine comparable to the nicotine obtained from smoking (Russel et al. 1981; Holm et al. 1992). Snuff has yet to be linked to any cancers, but, as it does contain known carcinogenic chemicals, it should not be seen as a completely safe alternative to smoking.

Those looking for an effective, natural, and safe way to suppress their appetite after using cannabis should look into drinking green tea. It may seem like a deceptively simple solution, but several studies have now looked at and confirmed the appetite-killing effectiveness of a green tea molecule called epigallocatechin gallate (Kao, Hiipakka, and Liao 2000; Sayama et all. 2000; Rains, Agarwal, and Maki 2011).

Of particular interest to the current discussion is a 2015 paper published in the *Journal of Clinical Biochemistry and Nutrition* (Song et al.) which found that green tea caused the release of appetite-suppressant hormones in the intestines. Since cannabis also works on the gut in order to stimulate the appetite, green tea may be able to provide a balancing effect.

The internet is replete with tips for suppressing the munchies, such as drinking a lot of water or eating a meal beforehand. While these tips may work for some people, they aren't consistent with what we know about how the munchies are caused. The suggestions given above are specifically formulated with known causes of the munchies in mind, intended to counteract the fact that cannabis enhances the senses and stimulates certain neurons and enzymes. Finding out what works for you may take some trial and error; it's sure to be a fun experience nevertheless.